DILEMMAS IN YOUTH WORK AND YOUTH DEVELOPMENT PRACTICE

The fundamental aim of youth work is to build trusting and mutually respectful relationships with young people, creating transformative experiences for young people in formal and informal spaces outside of homes and schools. These complex and multidimensional situations mean that the day-to-day work of youth workers is full of dilemmas, pitting moral, developmental, motivational, organizational, and other concerns against each other.

By showing how different youth workers respond to a variety of such dilemmas, this authentic text makes visible youth workers' unique knowledge and skills, and explores how to work with challenging situations – from the everyday to the extraordinary. Beginning by setting out a framework for dilemma resolution, it includes a number of narrative-based chapters in which youth workers describe and reflect on dilemmas they have faced, the knowledge and experiences they brought to bear on them, and alternative paths they could have taken. Each chapter closes with a discussion from the literature about themes raised in the chapter, an analysis of the dilemma and a set of overarching discussion questions designed to have readers compare and contrast the cases, consider what they would do in the situation, and reflect on their own practice.

Teaching us a great deal about the norms, conventions, continuities, and discontinuities of youth work, this practical book reveals essential dimensions of the profession and contributes to a practice-based theoretical foundation of youth work.

Laurie Ross is an Associate Professor of Community Development and Planning in the Department of International Development, Community and Environment at Clark University in Worcester, MA. She teaches on the Community Development and Planning Master's program and directs Clark's Certificate Program in Youth Work Practice. She engages in collaborative action and research with community partners on issues such as youth and gang violence, youth homelessness, and youth worker professional education.

Shane Capra is the Youth Program Coordinator and Co-op Incubation Coordinator at the Worcester Roots Project. He received his Master's in Community Development and Planning at Clark University in 2013. His final Master's paper is entitled "Re-orienting the map: exploring dilemma-based competency in social justice youth development."

Lindsay Carpenter is a Career Counselor with Job Corps, whose youth work has focused on young women and violence prevention. She received her Master's in Community Development and Planning at Clark University in 2011. Her final Master's paper is entitled "A framework to analyze youth workers' response to risky behavior: considerations of youth worker skill and organizational capacity."

Julia Hubbell is a Middle School Network Liaison within the Cambridge Public Schools where she creates awareness and connects young people to out-of-school-time (OST) opportunities. Her professional background has been with youth in urban areas where she has held roles in schools as an educator and also in OST settings as a youth worker. She received her Master's in Community Development and Planning at Clark University in 2012. Her final Master's paper is entitled "Dilemmas in youth work: a journey toward developing expertise."

Kathrin Walker is an Associate Professor and Specialist in Youth Work Practice at the University of Minnesota Extension Center for Youth Development. Her research explores the dilemmas that practitioners face in their everyday work with young people and their strategies for addressing these challenges.

DILEMMAS IN YOUTH WORK AND YOUTH DEVELOPMENT PRACTICE

Laurie Ross, Shane Capra, Lindsay Carpenter, Julia Hubbell and Kathrin Walker

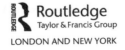

Routledge
Taylor & Francis Group

LONDON AND NEW YORK

First published 2016
by Routledge
2 Park Square, Milton Park, Abingdon, Oxon OX14 4RN

and by Routledge
711 Third Avenue, New York, NY 10017

Routledge is an imprint of the Taylor & Francis Group, an informa business

© 2016 L. Ross, S. Capra, L. Carpenter, J. Hubbell, and K. Walker

British Library Cataloguing-in-Publication Data
A catalogue record for this book is available from the British Library

Library of Congress Cataloging in Publication Data
Ross, Laurie.
Dilemmas in youth work and youth development practice / written by Laurie Ross, Shane Capra, Lindsay Carpenter, Julia Hubbell and Kathrin Walker. -- 1 Edition.
pages cm
Includes bibliographical references and index.
1. Youth workers--United States. 2. Employee motivation--United States. 3. Career development--United States. I. Title.
HV1431.R667 2015
362.7023'73--dc23
2015004108

ISBN: 978-1-138-84395-0 (hbk)
ISBN: 978-1-138-84396-7 (pbk)
ISBN: 978-1-315-73073-8 (ebk)

Typeset in Bembo
by Saxon Graphics Ltd, Derby

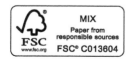

Printed and bound by CPI Group (UK) Ltd, Croydon, CR0 4YY

CONTENTS

BOXES, FIGURES AND TABLES

ACKNOWLEDGEMENTS

We offer our deep gratitude to the youth workers who contributed their stories to this book. You inspire us and we are thrilled that others will be able to learn from your knowledge, experience, and approach to youth work. While we can't acknowledge you by name, know that you are advancing the critically important field of youth work.

We also want to thank Todd Logan. The Seymour N. Logan Faculty Fellowship that his family provided catalyzed this project.

AUTHOR BIOGRAPHIES

Laurie Ross is an Associate Professor of Community Development and Planning in the Department of International Development, Community and Environment at Clark University in Worcester, MA. She teaches on the Community Development and Planning Master's program and directs Clark's Certificate Program in Youth Work Practice. She engages in collaborative action and research with community partners on issues such as youth and gang violence, youth homelessness, and youth worker professional education.

Shane Capra is the Youth Program Coordinator and Co-op Incubation Coordinator at the Worcester Roots Project. He received his Master's in Community Development and Planning at Clark University in 2013. His final Master's paper is entitled "Re-orienting the map: exploring dilemma-based competency in social justice youth development."

Lindsay Carpenter is a Career Counselor with Job Corps whose youth work has focused on young women and violence prevention. She received her Master's in Community Development and Planning at Clark University in 2011. Her final Master's paper is entitled "A framework to analyze youth workers' response to risky behavior: considerations of youth worker skill and organizational capacity."

Julia Hubbell is a Middle School Network Liaison within the Cambridge Public Schools where she creates awareness and connects young people to out-of-school-time (OST) opportunities. Her professional background has been with youth in urban areas where she has held roles in schools as an educator and also in OST settings as a youth worker. She received her Master's in Community Development and Planning at Clark University in 2012. Her final Master's paper is entitled "Dilemmas in youth work: a journey toward developing expertise."

Kathrin Walker is an Associate Professor and Specialist in Youth Work Practice at the University of Minnesota Extension Center for Youth Development. Her research explores the dilemmas that practitioners face in their everyday work with young people and their strategies for addressing these challenges.

1

BECOMING A YOUTH WORKER

Introduction: becoming a youth worker

The fundamental aim of youth work is to build trusting and mutually respectful relationships with young people. Youth workers create safe environments for children and teens to connect with supportive adults and to avoid violence in their neighborhoods and homes. They help young people to develop knowledge and skills in a variety of areas including academics, athletics, leadership, civics, the arts, health and well-being, and career exploration. Youth workers guide those harmed by oppressive community conditions such as racism, sexism, ageism, homophobia, and classism through a process of healing. In short, youth workers create transformative experiences for young people in formal and informal spaces, generally outside of homes and schools.

This work is not easy. The day-to-day life of youth workers is full of challenges and dilemmas that require deliberation and consideration of the merits of different possible actions. These situations are complex and multidimensional. They often pit moral, developmental, motivational, organizational, and other concerns against each other. Even the most experienced youth workers encounter situations that require them to balance competing goals and demands with the needs of youth (Larson and Walker, 2010). Yet in our research, practice, and teaching, we have found that highly effective youth workers are regularly able to size up situations and have a repertoire of effective responses. Unlike novices who can get stuck in determining a course of action and get sidetracked by a desire to be liked by the youth, experts steadfastly keep young people's interests and well-being at the center of their analysis and actions.

How does one become an expert youth worker? Are some people just born for this work? Is expertise developed and honed through experience on the job? Is there a role for professional education in the cultivation of the knowledge, skills, and disposition needed for transformative youth work? This book is aimed at providing some fodder to explore and begin to answer these questions for aspiring, novice, and even experienced youth workers. Through telling actual youth worker dilemma stories, we illustrate how youth workers navigate and figure out what to do in the face of difficult situations that involve competing priorities including the interests of youth, the youth organization, families, and communities. We focus on the types of knowledge and thought processes as well as the abilities to act and reflect that are required to resolve complex dilemmas of practice. Youth worker stories reveal that the types of knowledge and skills most often drawn upon in the resolution of dilemmas tend not to be those that are being focused on in efforts to professionalize the field of youth work in the United States. Much of the current research into youth worker practice is rooted in the standardization of conditions for positive youth development. While this is an important area of study, it often creates a set of goals for youth workers rather than an effective means of honing skills or navigating the daily tumult of working with young people.

The dilemmas in this book arose largely in urban settings in the northeast region of the United States and/or with youth with special needs. They focus on forging relationships with youth; setting high expectations for youth while acknowledging the realities of their day-to-day lives; managing groups; maintaining boundaries; handling incidents of violence and fights; addressing youth drug use; negotiating youth's gang involvement; and countering oppressive societal forces facing youth. This book is not meant to be read as a "how to" guide, and the dilemma stories are not meant to be prescriptive. We are not claiming that the youth workers in this book necessarily did the right or wrong thing in each case. Rather, we make visible how youth workers with varying degrees of experience, personal knowledge, and education approach a variety of dilemmas.

Before we present a dilemma-based approach to understanding and cultivating youth worker expertise, we tell the story that provided the initial inspiration to write this book. The story in Box 1.1 was first told in a university class on youth work that consisted of aspiring, novice, and experienced youth workers. We further developed the story with follow-up interviews with Jacob, one of the featured youth workers.[1]

BOX 1.1 "YOUTH WORK IS JUST COMMON SENSE"— JACOB, VETERAN YOUTH WORKER

We had just spent almost an hour discussing two particularly challenging situations in class. One case involved a youth worker's struggle about whether he should call the police when he was told a young person in his youth center had a gun. The other involved a different youth worker's decision to call Child Protective Services after hearing and seeing evidence of abuse on one of the children in her program. By the end of this intense discussion, the class understood and agreed with the actions both youth workers took. Jacob, a youth worker with over 20 years of experience, then made the statement: "Well, youth work is just common sense."

As the instructor, I found Jacob's remark to be pretty surprising. The conversations about these two situations had been extremely nuanced. It was apparent that both youth workers possessed a deep understanding of family dynamics, youth development, the juvenile justice system, the importance of working in teams, and how to negotiate between organizational rules and standards and doing what is best for the young people. The dialogue made explicit the youth workers' unique knowledge, experiences, and thought processes that guided both of them to make what ultimately was an effective decision. I thought to myself: "How could this possibly all be 'common sense'?"

I found Jacob's comment to be even more interesting in light of a discussion about another challenge that was raised in class. Sue—a white college student—had shared a story concerning her high school mentee who was African American. Her mentee admitted to her that she did not want to go to college. Sue could relate to ambivalence about college. She had left her first university after one semester and, despite knowing higher education opens up many opportunities, she did not like to accept that attending college determined one's success in life. Sue knew she should tell her mentee about the importance of higher education, but she also thought it would be helpful for her mentee to hear how she had worked through her own ambivalence. However, issues of race, class, and privilege flooded her mind. She was paralyzed in the moment about how to respond. She was afraid to overstep boundaries and she decided it wasn't her place to tell her mentee what to do and what path to take. In class, Sue expressed that she was dissatisfied with her response but wasn't sure what else she should have done.

Looking at these situations together is enlightening. On the one hand, we have two very experienced youth workers handling life or death situations with a third experienced youth worker summarizing their responses as 'common sense.' On the other hand, we have a novice youth worker who is trying to help a young person through a struggle similar to one she had recently gone through, but is unable find a satisfactory response to the situation. If youth work was just common sense, we would have thought this would have kicked in for the latter case—but clearly it did not.

The juxtaposition of these stories shows that expert youth workers respond to complex youth problems in a way that *seems* like common sense. Expert youth workers appraise situations, formulate plans of action, enact the plans, and upon reflection—either alone or with others—conclude that they make effective decisions more times than not. It would seem that framing youth work as common sense grossly simplifies what expert youth workers do and diminishes the rich personal and professional knowledge they possess about youth development and culture, and how to read a situation.

If this knowledge is so rich then we are left to wonder why Jacob minimized his own practice. Why do youth workers tend to diminish the importance of their work? Why is there a feeling on the part of many youth workers that their work and role is misunderstood and unvalued by the larger community—particularly when compared to other youth-serving fields, such as teaching and social work? Through follow-up interviews with Jacob, we learned that he wonders: "Are we seen as glorified babysitters? *Do people understand that we develop youth?!*"

When pushed a bit more, Jacob suggests his expertise comes from growing up in the same neighborhood as the youth he works with now, being mentored by older youth workers, and his ability to study people and learn fast. When he looks at his 20 plus years in the field, he is convinced that he has acquired the knowledge at least equivalent to sitting through 4 years of college. Yet when he looks at his status, his workload, and the personal sacrifices he has had to make to do the work that he absolutely loves, he is convinced that his organization is benefiting from his lack of formal education:

> At the end of the day, we all want to feel as if we have been compensated adequately for the amount of effort you give. Because in most cases these organizations are not equipped to pay top dollar to bring in the degree-carrying "educated" person, they find themselves with heavy staff turnover waiting for a "Jacob" to emerge in their program.

Jacob feels that because he doesn't have his degree, he must continue to impress and improve. He doesn't want to see a "ceiling" hit him. At the same time, perhaps to justify his position and level of compensation to himself, Jacob constructs his youth work practice as "common sense."

Youth worker professional identity and education in the United States

Jacob's internal struggles are understandable. In the United States, youth work lacks many of the characteristics that by conventional standards would define it as a profession or its workers as professionals (Anderson-Nathe, 2010; Fusco, 2011, 2012; Phelan, 2005; VeLure Roholt and Rana, 2011). A profession can be defined as an occupational group that claims a distinctive body of knowledge and whose members practice competently, with accountability, and contribute to the development of the profession's knowledge base (Fusco, 2013; Higgs *et al.*, 2001). Cusick further elaborates that competence in a field is signified by practitioners "achieving appropriate standards in their understanding and application of specialized knowledge and skill" (2001: 91). VeLure Roholt and Rana argue that youth work in the United States lacks these characteristics: "[t]here are multiple competing definitions, disciplinary frames, and desired outcomes" (2011: 321). The lack of a core body of knowledge, common definitions, and standards of practice makes it challenging to define youth work as a profession and to identify characteristics that are associated with youth worker expertise (Walker *et al.*, 2009; Walker and Walker, 2011). Nonetheless, while professional identity is at least in part associated with the acquisition of formally recognized qualifications such as college and advanced degrees, there has been acknowledgement in many fields that achieving expertise requires more than a degree (Schön, 1990). Higgs *et al.* claim that professional expertise in human services "resides in practice wisdom and practice artistry" (2001: 4).

The youth development field has developed a rich evidence base about the features of settings that promote positive youth development (Eccles and Gootman, 2002). Ideals such as "clear and consistent structure and appropriate supervision," "supportive relationships," and "support for efficacy and mattering" have been correlated with positive youth outcomes in many program evaluations. In order to develop a workforce that is able to operationalize these ideals, the field has begun to articulate the essential knowledge, skills, and behaviors—also known as competencies—that youth workers should possess (Akiva, 2005; Astroth *et al.*, 2004; Vance, 2010). It is difficult to refute that youth workers should be able to do things such as "understand and apply basic child and adolescent development principles"; "communicate and develop positive relationships with youth"; "demonstrate the attributes and qualities of a positive role model"; and "adapt, facilitate, and evaluate age-appropriate activities with and for the group."

The challenge comes in applying these principles in the day-to-day practice of youth work. Youth workers often find themselves in situations that are comprised of multidimensional, intersecting systems that are different for each individual and, in turn, contribute to the quality of the relationships and activities that occur in youth development spaces (Larson *et al.*, 2009). As Larson and Walker (2010) have discussed, the principles and competencies are guideposts but the path to get to each guidepost is anything but straightforward, especially when the principles and competencies come into conflict when handling a particular situation. Bessant (2011: 62) further elaborates on limitations of focusing on the acquisition of competencies alone:

> Competency-based training can produce highly proficient technicians possessing both novice and beginning level capacities who are able to follow instructions. It does not do so well if we are looking for reflexive and critical professionals able to decide when rules need to be adapted or broken.

In short, most of the existing literature on youth work and youth development more broadly does not offer a guide to understanding the day-to-day practice of youth workers and how to navigate complex dilemmas.

Alternatively, an *expertise* frame focuses on the successful application of knowledge and experience in context. Anderson-Nathe has discussed expertise in problem resolution as "a professional's ability to unite theory and specialized practice across unique circumstances" and frames professionalism in terms of the workers' ability to "encounter a scenario, assess its content, select the appropriate theoretical foundation for interpreting it, and then build a grounded response" (2010: 21). Walker and Gran have said that in the face of everyday dilemmas, expert youth workers "orchestrate multiple competencies into a full range of behaviors necessary for effective practice" (2010: 3). As Walker and Walker highlight, "it is not just about going through the motions, but having ongoing opportunities to work at addressing some of the most difficult problems in one's field with coaching, questioning and critical reflection" (2011: 44). Expertise requires a far more complex process that combines and blends different types of knowledge and skills in context-specific ways. This dynamic process allows youth workers to read and understand people and situations in order to resolve the everyday and extraordinary dilemmas of practice.

This book reveals important dimensions of youth worker expertise and what it accomplishes through the telling of rich and illustrative dilemma stories. Dilemma stories in which youth workers explain how they analyzed situations and those involved, how they interpreted what was happening, how they weighed their response options, and how they implemented and evaluated their responses provide a unique glimpse into youth worker expertise. A focus on dilemma stories complicates the current privileging of propositional or scientific knowledge in the training of youth workers and, by extension, the competency approach to youth worker professional education that is dominant in the United States. Through these stories, we quickly see that youth worker praxis isn't an either/or—competencies or expertise. Mastery of youth work competencies is unquestionably a foundation of good practice, but it isn't sufficient for becoming an expert youth worker. By featuring the role of reflection in the process of resolving complex dilemmas, we situate youth workers as the creators of youth work praxis or practice-theories. This process helps to recast youth workers' tacit knowledge—or what Jacob referred to as "common sense"—into a practice-theory of youth work. Youth worker knowledge and praxis can form the foundation of an alternative model of youth worker professional education, as proposed in this book.

Making youth worker knowledge and practice visible through dilemma stories

Ask youth workers about their job and invariably they will tell you a story. The story may be about that one youth who has stayed in their heart for years and years or that particular incident that they wish they could do over. Youth worker stories are almost always very interesting and entertaining, but they are also powerful learning tools because they convey their knowledge, skills, and overall approach to the work. Stories are great teaching and learning tools because they convey human experience in ways other texts do not (Bruner, 1991). Narratives give voice to the marginalized by retaining their accounts intact and in their own words (Eastmond, 2007). This attribute of narratives is particularly relevant to youth workers, who tend to be invisible as actors in youth development research and policy discussions.

Bruner has said that "to be worth telling, a tale must be about how an implicit canonical script has been breached, violated, or deviated from in a manner to do violence to … the 'legitimacy' of the canonical script" (1991: 11). Youth worker dilemma stories are breaches to theories of youth development. For example, a foundational strand of positive youth development theory is youth's need for physical and psychological safety (Eccles and Gootman, 2002). Yet in the day-to-day practice of youth workers, what it means to create an environment that maintains physical and psychological safety is anything but straightforward. Several chapters in this book illustrate the balancing act that can be required to maintain safety. For example, in Chapter 9 we learn more about Jacob and another youth worker Ricardo and how they both handled the potential for gun violence in their organizations. Jacob and Ricardo describe their attempts to balance the safety and well-being of the potential shooters, other youth and staff at the organizations, and members of the larger community. These gun narratives, because they are extreme, are particularly effective in illustrating the importance of personal and practice knowledge in youth workers' attempts to analyze situations and those involved, interpret what is happening, weigh their response options, and implement and evaluate their responses (Ross, 2012). These types of stories complicate what it means to maintain an environment that promotes physical and psychological safety, while providing a unique glimpse into youth worker expertise.

Another foundational feature of positive youth development theory is the need to provide young people with opportunities for skill building. In Chapter 4, we explore stories about how two youth workers had to make decisions about whether to uphold, bend, or break program rules and expectations to ensure young people gained maximum benefit from their programs. Melinda has to decide whether or not to allow a young person in her group to stay on the dance team even though she is failing in school. Loren struggles with whether to allow a group of extremely disruptive students back into her high school equivalency diploma class. Again, the principle of providing young people with opportunities for skill building is straightforward and not controversial. The challenge is how to do that in the context of day-to-day practice. Hearing how youth workers such as Jacob, Ricardo, Melinda, and Loren attempt to resolve these "breaches" provides insight into how useful current theories are for day-to-day practice, and opens space for youth worker practice-theories to influence the field.

Ecological Dilemma Resolution model

Eight chapters in this book feature youth worker dilemma stories. Each story is an individual youth worker's account of his/her approach to resolving a particular dilemma. When read as a collection, we can learn a great deal about the norms, conventions, continuities, and discontinuities of youth work and, by extension, what it means to put youth development theory into practice. The accumulation of youth worker dilemma stories reveals essential dimensions of this profession and contributes to a practice-based theoretical foundation of youth work. We offer a framework that makes youth workers' practice-theories visible and explicit. We call this framework the Ecological Dilemma Resolution (EDR) model. Further elaborated in Chapter 2, the EDR model has three interrelated components: 1) forms of knowledge, 2) a structured dilemma resolution process, and 3) the application of ecological intelligence.

Knowledge

Knowledge *about* youth development theory, research, and approaches to youth work (also known as propositional knowledge) is the predominant learning outcome of most formal approaches to youth worker professional education in the United States. The ways youth workers in this book resolve dilemmas, however, suggest that formal knowledge alone is inadequate to explain how they *know what to do* in very challenging situations. The EDR model makes visible other forms of knowledge youth workers draw on, namely personal and practice knowledge (Higgs *et al.*, 2001; Hildreth and VeLure Roholt, 2013). These other forms of knowledge have been understudied by youth development researchers and largely overlooked by policy-makers and program developers. The chapters in this book show how youth workers bring personal and practice knowledge into their work as they resolve complex dilemmas. The chapters also guide readers on ways to activate their own personal and practice knowledge.

Dilemma resolution process

In comparing novices and experienced youth workers, Walker and Larson (2012) discovered distinct patterns in how experts approach and resolve complex dilemmas. Expert youth workers carefully appraise dilemmas in ways that generate many possible solutions. They anticipate possible outcomes of various solutions and are strategic in choosing the course of action with the most potential for favorable outcomes. They also tend to reflect on the effectiveness of their choice of actions in a way that guides their responses to future situations.

Reading dilemma stories in which youth workers explain how they analyzed a situation and those involved, how they interpreted what was happening, how they weighed their response options, and how they implemented and evaluated their responses guides youth workers toward a more deliberative way of thinking about youth work. Working with cases helps youth workers develop the patterns of thought needed when they are confronted with dilemmas on the job.

A second dimension that differentiated experts from novices in Larson and Walker's (2010) work was that the experts were much more likely to craft youth-centered responses to dilemmas. Their research found that a youth-centered response has the following four attributes:

- engaging directly with youth;
- turning the dilemma into an opportunity for youth's development;

- incorporating youth into the solution or response to the situation; and
- advocating on behalf of youth as well as teaching youth to advocate for themselves.

In Chapters 3 through 10 we highlight the ways the youth workers use youth-centered responses in their dilemmas.

Ecological intelligence

By analyzing what expert youth workers do when confronted with complex dilemmas of practice, we also have come to see the value of bringing an ecological lens into this work (Bronfenbrenner, 1979). Ecologically informed analysis can help youth workers understand interactions between youth and their environments and the ways identities, values, beliefs, practices, roles, and relationships intersect within and across multiple settings in the context of power differences (Derksen, 2010; Larson and Walker, 2010). The stories from the more experienced youth workers in this book suggest that they have what Walker and Larson (2012) have called "ecological intelligence" because they intuitively engage in ecological analysis when confronted by complex dilemmas. The reflection questions and recommended activities at the end of each chapter are meant to guide readers in their development of ecological intelligence.

Ecological Dilemma Resolution model summary

Chapters 3 through 10 apply the EDR model to youth worker dilemma stories. These chapters provide deeper insight into how different youth workers respond to a variety of dilemmas and in turn reveal what it means to *be* a youth worker. The application of the EDR model informs professional education by revealing the skills, attitudes, and knowledge needed to be a transformative youth worker. More than *learning about* effective practice, the EDR model advances a "dilemma-based pedagogy" that helps *improve* youth work by inviting readers to use the model to:

- activate their personal and practice knowledge;
- develop patterns of thought needed to conduct comprehensive yet rapid analysis of dilemma situations; and
- recognize and be able to navigate the ecological complexity of youth work dilemmas.

Where did the dilemma stories in this book come from?

The dilemma stories in this book come from a multi-year classroom-based action research project aimed at understanding how youth workers resolve complex problems of practice (Ross, 2012).[2] The university course on youth work enrolls both traditional students and community youth workers. All of the students in the course are involved in youth work through employment, an internship, or a volunteer opportunity.

Dilemma stories are the primary texts used in the course. The original set of dilemma stories came from in-depth interviews Ross conducted with 15 youth workers. When she started the project, she had been engaged in youth work for over ten years. She used her youth work networks to identify highly regarded and experienced youth workers. Of the 15, 8 were male, 3 were white, 5 were black, and 7 were Latino. Their average age was 36 and the average number of years on the job was just over 15, with a range of 5 to over 40. Ten were community "insiders" in that they grew up in the city where they work and attended youth programs there. The interviews, which took an hour on average to conduct, inquired about their path to youth work, a typical work day, stories about specific dilemmas they faced, how they resolved those dilemmas, and their future aspirations. In several instances, Ross conducted follow-up interviews to capture more details about particular stories. These interviews were audio recorded with the youth workers' consent and transcribed. The transcriptions were used to construct the dilemma case studies in this book; language and flow were altered to enhance the understandability of the story, but we attempted to keep the narratives as close to the youth workers' own words as possible.

Dilemma case studies are also the final product of this university course. Over the semester, students have a number of assignments that culminate into a final dilemma case study. First, students write their youth worker autobiography in which they are instructed to describe critical incidents that led them to this field and that keep them committed to it. They are asked to think intentionally about where their youth work knowledge and skills come from. Students are also required to keep guided dilemma journals. Students are asked to provide a deep description of challenges they are facing, to include the outcomes of their actions, and to reflect on how they handled the dilemmas. Students share journal entries in class to hear how others would handle the problem as well as to provide an opportunity to analyze the causes and structure of the problems. For the final assignment, students choose one dilemma to develop into a full case study. They integrate insights from their autobiography into the case. They are required to suggest readings to accompany the case, and to design a training activity. Capra, Carpenter, and Hubbell—all former students of this class—went a step further and used the dilemma framework to conduct their master's research. To date, we have collected and analyzed hundreds of youth worker dilemma stories, with roughly 35 of them turned into full case studies.

The stories we chose to include in this book do a particularly good job of illustrating the three components of the EDR model: 1) forms of knowledge; 2) steps in the Dilemma Resolution Cycle; and 3) the utilization of "ecological intelligence." They highlight areas where both novices and experts get stuck and invite readers to consider what they would do in their own practice if confronted with such a dilemma. Because the action research project and the class were heavily influenced by Kate Walker's research and her writing on the dilemmas of youth work practice, we invited her to help identify crosscutting themes and explore the implications for youth worker professional development; this is provided in Chapter 11.

How to use this book

This book makes visible the practice wisdom and artistry of a diverse group of novice and expert youth workers. We explain and validate the sophisticated, actionable knowledge that these youth workers bring to their work, creating a space for youth workers' voices and experiences to advance the field. Central to this book is understanding how one *becomes* a youth worker—not in a "how to" sense, but rather how one develops the knowledge, skills, and disposition to work with young people relationally with the goal of mutual transformation.

Our aim is not only to make visible and validate youth worker knowledge, however. Ultimately, this book can help novice and experienced youth workers advance their own practice. Chapter 2 more fully develops the EDR model. We provide the theoretical foundations of the model including youth worker knowledge and expertise, the dilemma resolution process, ecological intelligence, and reflection in- and on-practice. We demonstrate how the EDR model can be used to strengthen youth workers' practice through a thorough analysis of Kelli's dilemma story (see Table 2.1). Chapter 2 concludes with exercises we recommend readers complete before reading the dilemma chapters.

Chapters 3–10 are organized around a particular type of youth worker dilemma (see Box 1.2). Each chapter includes one or two dilemma stories and provides background information about the youth worker(s) and her/his organization(s). We present the learning objectives of the case and then offer a detailed presentation of how the youth worker(s) approached the dilemma and his/her reflections on the outcome. Each of these chapters contains a section called "Unpacking the dilemma," in which we use the EDR model to analyze the types of knowledge the youth workers used in their dilemma resolution process. We use the EDR model to highlight the youth workers' internal struggles and where he/she may have gotten stuck.

Also in "Unpacking the dilemma," we provide "Reflecting on practice" questions designed to have readers compare and contrast the cases, consider what they would do in the situation, and reflect on their own practice. Ultimately, these questions are meant to help readers develop the "ecological intelligence" needed to effectively resolve youth work dilemmas. Youth workers can answer these questions on their own, or they could be used by faculty or trainers to generate group discussion. Each of these chapters concludes with a section called "Digging deeper: applying the dilemma to your work." This section includes several activities that can be done on one's own or in groups of youth workers. While this is the general format for each chapter, there is some variation across the stories. For example, we intentionally varied the amount of biographical information provided in order to consider the importance of the youth workers' own life stories in how they resolve complex dilemmas. Chapter 11 concludes the book by examining crosscutting themes and discussing implications for youth worker professional education. Our hope for this book is to make youth workers' practice-theories visible in a way that contributes to a transformative form of youth worker professional education in the United States.

BOX 1.2 DILEMMA CHAPTERS AND SAMPLE LEARNING OBJECTIVES

Chapter 3 Navigating inexperience: how reflection guides practice for a novice youth worker
- Developing relationships with mentors and youth
- Thinking on your feet

Chapter 4 Balancing high expectations, program structure, and youth realities: making kids fit the program or the program fit the kids
- Recognizing when personal triggers or disappointments in youth performance cloud judgment
- Knowing when to be flexible with program rules and standards to ensure all youth can benefit from the program

Chapter 5 Balancing conflicting values from home, a youth organization, and the community: keeping youth well-being at the center of youth work
- Keeping youth's needs and well-being at the center of a youth worker's practice
- Drawing on resources and networks outside of one's organization

Chapter 6 Youth worker and organizational responses to risky behavior and dangerous situations
- Thinking on your feet in high-stress situations
- Knowing and using your organization's policies

Chapter 7 Balancing youth privacy with the youth worker's need for information: the importance of organizational support in dilemma resolution
- Understanding the need for "plan B" when tried-and-true strategies are not working
- Utilizing appropriate lines of communication within an organization to resolve dilemmas

Chapter 8 Activating personal knowledge to balance the needs of high-risk youth with the safety of others in the program
- Balancing the needs of a few "high-risk" youth with the safety of the overall program population
- Using personal and professional networks to evaluate and resolve a dilemma

---

**Chapter 9 "When I heard who it was, I knew it wasn't a real gun":
"reading" the context to maintain safety**

- Rapidly reading potentially dangerous situations
- Using reflection as a tool to transform personal experience into practice knowledge

**Chapter 10 "Do they think we're not in charge?" Addressing
dilemmas that arise in a Social Justice Youth Development approach**

- Being proactive in negotiating relationships with partner organizations
- Channeling anger and frustration into creating teachable moments for youth

---

Notes

1 All names of individuals, groups, organizations, and locations have been changed to protect the identity and confidentiality of the youth worker and the youth development organization.
2 This project went through Human Subjects review and was approved by the Institutional Review Board at Ross's university. All of the youth workers involved and students in the class were aware of the scholarly and applied aspects of the project.

References

Akiva, T. (2005). Turning training into results: The new Youth Program Quality Assessment. *High/Scope ReSource*, Fall/Winter, 21–4.

Anderson-Nathe, B. (2010). *Youth workers, stuckness, and the myth of supercompetence: Not knowing what to do*. London: Routledge.

Astroth, K., Garza, P., and Taylor, B. (2004). Getting down to business: Defining competencies for entry-level youth workers. *New Directions for Youth Development, 104*, 25–37.

Bessant, J. (2011). Youth work and the education of professional practitioners in Australia. In D. Fusco (Ed.), *Advancing youth work: Current trends, critical questions*. New York: Routledge (pp. 52–68).

Bronfenbrenner, U. (1979). *The ecology of human development: Experiments by nature and design*. Cambridge, MA: Harvard University Press.

Bruner, J. (1991). The narrative construction of reality. *Critical Inquiry, 18*(1), 1–21.

Cusick, A. (2001). Personal frames of reference in professional practice. In J. Higgs and A. Titchen (Eds.), *Practice knowledge and expertise in the health professions*. Oxford: Butterworth-Heinemann (pp. 91–5).

Derksen, T. (2010). The influence of ecological theory in child and youth care: A review of the literature. *International Journal of Child, Youth and Family Studies, 1*(3/4), 326–39.

Eastmond, M. (2007). Stories as lived experience: Narratives in forced migration research. *Journal of Refugee Studies, 20*(2), 248–64.

Eccles, J. and Gootman, J. (2002). *Community programs to promote youth development*. Washington, DC: National Academy Press.

Fusco, D. (2011). On becoming an academic profession. In D. Fusco (Ed.), *Advancing youth work: Current trends, critical questions*. New York: Routledge (pp. 111–26).

Fusco, D. (2012). Use of self in the context of youth work. *Child & Youth Services, 33*(1), 33–45.

Fusco, D. (2013). Is youth work being courted by the appropriate suitor? *Child & Youth Services, 34*(2), 196–209.

Higgs, J., Titchen, A., and Neville, V. (2001). Professional practice and knowledge. In J. Higgs and A. Titchen (Eds.), *Practice knowledge and expertise in the health professions.* Oxford: Butterworth-Heinemann (pp. 3–9).

Hildreth, R. and VeLure Roholt, R. (2013). Teaching and training civic youth workers: Creating spaces for reciprocal civic and youth development. In R. VeLure Roholt, M. Baizerman, and R. Hildreth (Eds.), *Civic youth work: Co-creating democratic youth spaces.* Chicago: Lyceum Books (pp. 151–9).

Larson, R. and Walker, K. (2010). Dilemmas of practice: Challenges to program quality encountered by youth program leaders. *American Journal of Community Psychology, 45*(3–4), 338–49.

Larson, R., Rickman, A., Gibbons, C., and Walker, K. (2009). Practitioner expertise: Creating quality within the daily tumble of events in youth settings. *New Directions for Youth Development, 121,* 71–88.

Phelan, J. (2005). Child and youth care education: The creation of articulate practitioners. *Child & Youth Care Forum, 34*(5), 347–55.

Ross, L. (2012). Disrupting borders: A case study in engaged pedagogy. *Michigan Journal of Community Service Learning, 19*(1), 58–68.

Schön, D. (1990). *Educating the reflective practitioner: Toward a new design for teaching and learning in the professions.* San Francisco: Jossey Bass.

Vance, F. (2010). A comparative analysis of competency frameworks for youth workers in the out-of-school time field. *Child & Youth Care Forum, 39*(6), 421–41.

VeLure Roholt, R. and Rana, S. (2011). Improving community-based youth work: An evaluation of an action research approach. *Child & Youth Services, 32*(4), 317–35.

Walker, J. and Walker, K. (2011). Establishing expertise in an emerging field. In D. Fusco (Ed.), *Advancing youth work: Current trends, critical questions.* New York: Routledge (pp. 39–51).

Walker, J., Gran, C., and Moore, D. (2009). *Once we know it, we can grow it: A framework for quality nonformal learning opportunities and youth work practice.* St. Paul, MN: University of Minnesota Extension Center for Youth Development.

Walker, K. and Gran, C. (2010). *Beyond core competencies: Practitioner expertise as a critical component of quality.* St. Paul, MN: University of Minnesota Extension Center for Youth Development.

Walker, K. and Larson, R. (2012). Youth worker reasoning about dilemmas encountered in practice: Expert-novice differences. *Journal of Youth Development, 7*(1), 5–23.

2

LEARNING TO "READ"

Cultivating ecological intelligence

Expert youth workers *appear* to have a magical ability to read young people's minds and understand their motivations and triggers. Not only can expert youth workers diagnose situations; their decisions about courses of action turn out to be effective more times than not. Expert youth workers make very complex situations look relatively easy to resolve, perhaps leading Jacob in Chapter 1 to chalk up his practice to "common sense." When we break down the way expert youth workers approach a wide range of dilemmas, however, we can see that while there might be a little magic going on, there is actually a rigorous art and science to youth work.

Expert youth workers are able to "read" people, actions, and contexts in order to formulate effective responses to dilemmas. "Ecological intelligence" appears to be a key factor in explaining how expert youth workers are able to do this. Ecological intelligence is deep, contextualized knowledge of youth culture and the systems that influence youth development. In their research distinguishing novice and expert youth workers, Walker and Larson (2012) found that novices were more likely to jump to solutions and apply context-free rules in their attempts to resolve dilemmas. The experts, on the other hand, demonstrated contextual sensitivity in their analysis of the multiple people, perspectives, and systems relevant to resolving a dilemma. Expert youth workers' ecological intelligence:

> appeared to involve, not solely knowledge of these different systems, but possession of elaborated mental models of how different systems worked and the leverage points for influencing them. These were evident in the experts more frequent formation of hypotheses about root causes of youth's or other people's behavior, hypotheses that, in real life situations, might help them better know what questions to ask or information to seek. These mental models were also evidence in the experts' greater engagement in forecasting

events, anticipating contingencies, and formulating decision trees that took these possible contingencies into account.

(Walker and Larson, 2012: 8)

Walker and Larson concluded that the experts' conceptual and operational understanding of varied systems allowed them to tailor their responses to dilemmas appropriately.

In the midst of dilemmas involving competing forces such as school, family, neighborhood, and peer group, ecologically intelligent youth workers are able to center the youth's interest and well-being. These youth workers rely on their understanding of neighborhoods, schools, and larger systems such as child welfare and juvenile justice as they decide how to handle complex dilemmas. Ecologically intelligent youth workers understand interactions between youth and their environments, and the ways identities, values, beliefs, practices, roles, and relationships intersect within and across multiple settings in the context of power differences (Bessant, 2011; Derksen, 2010; Larson and Walker, 2010). The stories from the more experienced youth workers in this book illustrate ecological intelligence in action.

This book advances a framework for the development of "ecological intelligence" in the ongoing professional education of youth workers. We call this framework the Ecological Dilemma Resolution (EDR) model. Developing the concepts introduced in Chapter 1, we define the EDR model in this chapter and apply it in Chapters 3 through 10. Through its application to youth worker dilemma stories, the EDR model makes youth worker knowledge and practice visible and shows how youth workers draw on ecological intelligence to read people, actions, and situations that allow them to resolve complex and ambiguous youth work dilemmas.

The Ecological Dilemma Resolution model

The objective of the EDR model is to facilitate the development of ecological intelligence in youth workers. The EDR model consists of two components: 1) youth worker knowledge and 2) a structured dilemma resolution process. Before we describe these two components, we provide a conceptual underpinning for ecological intelligence.

Ecological intelligence is grounded in Urie Bronfenbrenner's seminal work on the ecology of human development (Bronfenbrenner, 1979). The ecology of human development refers to the environments, relationships, and experiences that influence the development of young people and their families. Bronfenbrenner identified a set of interconnected, embedded systems that influence human development (see Figure 2.1). The first is the "microsystem"—or the young person's immediate environments, such as the family, the school, the youth development organization, the peer group, and the neighborhood. The developmental building blocks of microsystems are the activities, relationships, and roles that occur within them. The second is the "mesosystem"—or the

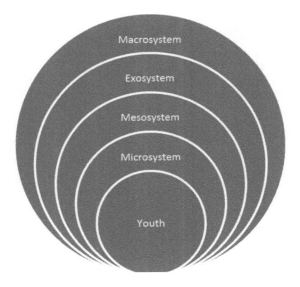

FIGURE 2.1 The ecology of human development

relationships among microsystems, including the structure and level of coherence in the connections between various microsystems, such as those between the family and the school or between the neighborhood and the peer group. The third is the "exosystem," defined as the contexts in which the child is not immediately present but which directly influence the microsystem, such as parents' employment situation and school board policies. The fourth is the "macrosystem," defined as the consistencies in the form and content of micro-, meso-, and exosystems at the level of the subculture or the culture as a whole. Political systems, gender norms, social constructions of race, and other broad socioeconomic dynamics shape the macrosystem, which in turn influences the extent to which given microsystems promote healthy development for subgroups of youth.

Figure 2.1 provides a relatively simple diagram of the idea of nested systems. Figure 2.2 is a more complex illustration that focuses on one of the foundational elements of a youth development organization microsystem—the relationship between the youth and the youth worker or, using Bronfenbrenner's terminology, the youth-youth worker dyad.

Figure 2.2 represents the nested set of ecological systems that influence the young person coming through the door of a local youth organization. An ecologically intelligent youth worker is mindful about how these influences shape a young person's behaviors and experiences on any given day. This youth worker is also aware of his or her own developmental ecology and how the interaction between their ecologies affects their relationship generally and the dilemma resolution process more specifically.

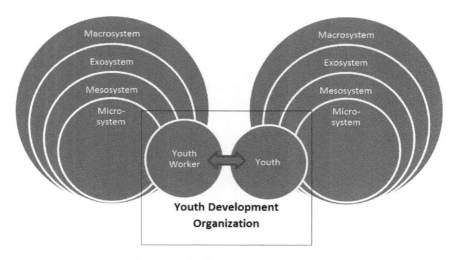

FIGURE 2.2 Youth–youth worker dyad

We now delve deeper into the two other components of the EDR model: multiple forms of knowledge and a structured dilemma resolution process. We examine the types of knowledge that undergird ecological intelligence. We also elaborate a structured process for youth workers to determine which ecological features are relevant in a particular dilemma.

Knowledge

Scholars who study professional expertise have identified categories of knowledge and abilities that are required to excel in particular fields (Ericsson *et al.*, 2006; Higgs and Bithell, 2001). In youth work, Hildreth and VeLure Roholt (2013) discuss how expertise is connected to the interplay of three forms of knowledge: propositional, practice (or professional craft), and personal (depicted in Figure 2.3). *Propositional knowledge* is formal knowledge about youth development theory, research, and approaches to youth work. Propositional knowledge is the predominant learning outcome of most higher education programs and other forms of professional education. Knowledge about topics such as youth development, group dynamics, and the child welfare system is necessary to be an effective youth worker. Yet, propositional knowledge alone is generally not sufficient to resolve complex dilemmas of practice (Bessant, 2011; Ord, 2014; Walker and Gran, 2010).

The second form of knowledge, *practice knowledge* (or *professional craft knowledge*), is rich practice knowledge accumulated by doing the work over time and having opportunities to reflect-on-practice (Emslie, 2009; Schön, 1990). Professional craft knowledge includes practical skills as well as the development of reasoning and judgment needed to make difficult decisions (Higgs and Bithell, 2001). Because professional knowledge is accumulated over time and on a case-by-case basis (sometimes through trial and error), it is difficult to quantify and label. It is knowledge that can only come from experience and cannot be *taught* in a traditional sense. It is often this professional knowledge of youth and youth work that can be mistaken for common sense; youth workers may not be cognizant that this practical learning is happening.

Finally, *personal knowledge* is knowledge "about oneself as a person and in relationship with others" (Higgs *et al.*, 2001: 5). This form of knowing requires "a solid *understanding* of the personal knowledge we carry with us into our practice" (Hildreth and VeLure Roholt, 2013: 153; emphasis added). The concept of "understanding" is stressed to connote that personal knowledge is not simply a matter of having had a collection of life experiences that may be similar to the youth's but, rather, that a youth worker has made meaning of her own life story— that she has engaged in self-reflection both to understand her own biases and preconceived notions about young people (Cusick, 2001) and to transform social learning from accumulated life experiences with formal education into actionable knowledge (Lave and Wenger, 1991).

Practitioner expertise involves not only universal propositional knowledge but also professional craft knowledge as well as reflective personal knowledge. Moreover, it involves what Aristotle called "phronesis" or prudent, practical wisdom about what is right and good. This type of contextual knowledge is central to youth work (Ord, 2014) and to making sound, ethical decisions when navigating challenging dilemmas like those explored in this book (Walker and Walker, 2011).

Reflection and metacognitive skills are critical in transforming these forms of knowledge into practical, actionable knowledge (Wood *et al.*, 2015). Fusco has stated that the use of self in youth work can be defined as "a nexus of interaction and activity that occurs intentionally, purposefully, and relationally in order to

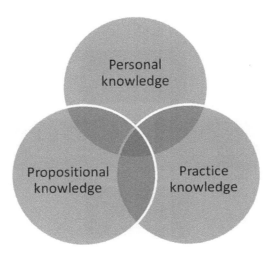

FIGURE 2.3 Forms of knowledge

bring about human change" (2012: 34) and involves "observing, listening, questioning, communicating, reflecting, acknowledging, accepting, empathy and self-awareness" (2012: 37). Krueger has described self-in-action in youth work in the following way:

> to understand a child's fear, sadness, loss, trauma, joy, for instance, workers have to be able to understand how they themselves experience these emotions so they can understand how their feelings influence their understanding of and contribute to their interactions with children.
>
> *(1997: 154)*

It is in knowing oneself that one can "know" and "be" with the young people. This is the heart of youth work expertise—the ability to use practical wisdom not only to build relationships with youth, but to engage and work relationally with young people in a range of contexts and on a vast array of issues (Fusco, 2012; Spence, 2008).

Structured dilemma resolution process

The second part of the EDR considers how youth workers apply this integrated and actionable knowledge to reading people, actions, and situations. Walker and Larson (2012) discovered distinct patterns in how expert youth workers approach and resolve complex dilemmas. These patterns break down into a four-part cycle of 1) problem recognition and appraisal, 2) plan formulation, 3) plan implementation, and 4) evaluation and reflection, as shown in Figure 2.4.

While this process appears straightforward, our analysis of dilemma stories shows that novices tend to get stuck during this Dilemma Resolution Cycle much more frequently than experts. Research on expertise in multiple fields has found that novices tend to be inefficient in the face of dilemmas and difficult decisions. They become easily overwhelmed by the complexity of "real life" because they have not

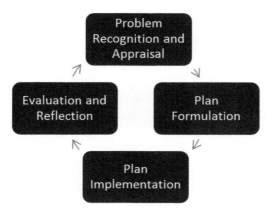

FIGURE 2.4 Structured dilemma resolution process

developed mental models that help them to recognize patterns in dilemmas and to work through problems of practice (Endsley, 2006). As a result, novices either get paralyzed into inaction or they jump to an easy explanation and solution that may not adequately address the problem.

Experts, on the other hand, are able to appraise multiple dimensions of a dilemma (Endsley, 2006). They consider visual and auditory cues, history, and the actions of others in the situation. Their thorough review allows the experts to generate many possible explanations for the problem. They sift through the information and determine which factors are most relevant. Based on their reading of the situation, they are able to formulate possible resolutions. They anticipate outcomes of various options and are strategic in choosing the course of action with the most potential for favorable outcomes. They also tend to reflect on the effectiveness of their choice of actions in a way that guides their responses to future situations (Larson and Walker, 2010). Depending on the type of dilemma, this process may need to occur either in a matter of seconds or over the course of several weeks or even months. Reflecting back on how one worked through the dilemma resolution process in a particular case helps the youth worker derive learning from experience, thereby building their knowledge base for future dilemmas (Wood *et al.*, 2015).

★★★

Figure 2.5 is a visual representation of the EDR model. To summarize, ecological intelligence is derived from personal, propositional, and practice knowledge that

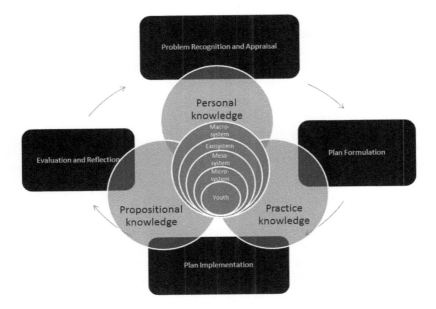

FIGURE 2.5 Ecological Dilemma Resolution model

has been activated through reflective, deliberative practice. Ecological intelligence informs the stages of the youth worker Dilemma Resolution Cycle: problem recognition, plan formulation, plan implementation, and reflection.

Youth worker dilemmas as text: using the Ecological Dilemma Resolution model to enhance practice

In their day-to-day practice, youth workers need to make their propositional, practice, and personal knowledge actionable. They have to be able to draw on theories of adolescent development, use critical thinking to understand ecological considerations, engage in creative problem-solving, and apply judgment in decision-making (Walker and Walker, 2011). While propositional knowledge has been codified into textbooks and training manuals, practice and personal knowledge often remains tacit. And even when youth workers have access to propositional knowledge, knowing how to use it in practice is often challenging.

Case studies have been used in other fields to make these forms of knowledge explicit, sharable, and actionable (Cianciolo *et al.*, 2006; Curry *et al.*, 2011; Walker and Walker, 2011). Real-world situations trigger learning; cases simulate reality in a way that forces students to exercise judgment, consider multiple options, think through implications of courses of action, and reflect on what they would do in that type of situation. Cases about challenging situations can help novices understand the complexities of practice. Cases encourage metacognition which is needed to improve day-to-day practice.

Reading youth worker dilemma case studies through the lens of the EDR model opens up rich professional education opportunities. We gain insight into how youth workers understand problems of practice and into their decision-making. We can see where youth workers tend to get "stuck" in the process of implementing possible solutions. Through an EDR-guided analysis of cases, youth workers begin to identify their own triggers and personal roadblocks. The model offers a structured way to work on real-world problems as well as a way to practice problem-solving from multiple perspectives, applying multiple considerations.

In Table 2.1, we provide an example of how to apply the EDR model to a youth worker dilemma story. In the left column, we present Kelli's dilemma. Kelli is a novice youth worker and college student. She has had a multi-year mentoring relationship with a middle school-aged girl named Jestina. In this dilemma story, Jestina reveals a personal concern to Kelli. Jestina's personal issue was quite familiar to Kelli as she had experienced something similar herself, yet she was unable to respond in a way that was satisfactory to either herself or Jestina. In the right column, we use the EDR model to analyze different dimensions of the dilemma. By applying the EDR model to the story, we begin to see the limitations of Kelli's ecological intelligence as well as opportunities for Kelli to improve her practice.

TABLE 2.1 Applying the Ecological Dilemma Resolution model

Kelli's dilemma	EDR analysis
At this point in my life, I consider myself a novice youth worker. I worked with youth as a camp counselor when I was 15, but that experience was pretty easy and fun. I have also worked in a residential program for youth. That wasn't as much fun. I found working with young people with serious emotional problems very challenging. I was in over my head there. When I started college, I got involved with a community-based mentoring program. I was a little hesitant at the start as I was anxious about working with youth in the city; but much to my relief, I felt an immediate connection with my mentee Jestina. The daily struggles she faced were on a scale I felt as though I could actually handle. <u>That was until Jestina told me she wanted to be skinnier.</u>	**Knowledge:** We get a glimpse into Kelli's prior experience in youth work, and the extent of her practice knowledge. **Problem Recognition:** The underlined text in the first paragraph is the first hint of the dilemma.
It was the beginning of the school year and I had just returned to campus. I had been in Vermont for the summer so I had not seen Jestina. When we did reconnect, I noticed that Jestina had altered her style from the year before. Her clothing was more mature and she was wearing makeup. Though I took notice of the changes, Jestina still seemed to be the shy and sweet girl I had gotten to know over the past couple of years. It was not until a few weeks into the semester that I realized Jestina's changes in appearance may be reflecting some more serious internal struggles. One day while Jestina was at my apartment helping bake cookies, she expressed her desire to lose weight. <u>For some reason the words "I want to be skinnier" hit more intensely than I ever would have thought. The moment she said it, I just froze. I was completely unsure how to handle the situation and the all too familiar struggle made my stomach drop.</u>	Kelli "reads" Jestina. She notices changes in her, but she doesn't consider the changes to be indicative of a problem and doesn't inquire about the changes. Kelli realizes that something about Jestina's struggle triggers her and clouds her judgment, making it difficult for her to react in a constructive and supportive way. She actually feels Jestina's struggle in her body, indicated by her statement: "the all too familiar struggle made my stomach drop."
I tried to find words as a jumbled stream of reactions ran through my mind. I didn't actually ask her why she wanted to lose weight; I assumed that I knew what she was going through. Initially, I wanted to contest what she just had shared. I wanted to tell her she was beautiful and that it was society that was ugly. But that not only felt incredibly hypocritical, it seemed like I would just be brushing the issue aside. There was a part of me that admitted that I already wondered whether Jestina might struggle with her weight, and at times I did worry a bit about her eating habits. *My growing awareness of the concept of food justice only really complicated my thought process, as I knew that accessibility and affordability of healthy food was more than likely an*	Kelli knows that Jestina does not have great eating habits and is a bit overweight. Kelli believes that Jestina's concern about her weight is justified. **Knowledge:** Italicized text suggests that her formal knowledge about food justice complicates rather than facilitates her ability to react to the problem. She is aware of larger systems that dictate food access; but this

TABLE 2.1 Continued

issue her family faced. Though my biggest concern in the moment was Jestina's self-esteem, it felt wrong to ignore the possibility that Jestina might eventually face health problems if her eating habits did not improve.

knowledge is not actionable. Kelli has not worked on how to integrate this formal knowledge into her practice.

After a few moments of fiddling with cookie dough and uncomfortable silence, I realized that there were useful recommendations I could make that seemed sensitive as well as appropriate. "Let's try to be more active when we hang out. And maybe we can even make healthy dinners at my house." I could tell Jestina was not completely satisfied with the suggestion but she did not press the issue any more. In retrospect, I fear I may have made her uncomfortable and discouraged her from sharing these feelings again. But in the moment, I was somewhat relieved. Ultimately we did follow through with the suggestions. We spent more time going for walks and playing basketball. Our plans to make healthy meals were only periodically feasible. I did feel some comfort with this, however, because Jestina shared with me that she often cooked dinner for her family.

Plan Formulation: Kelli breaks through her paralysis and decides to make suggestions about what they can do together that could address Jestina's concerns about her weight.

Plan Implementation: Once she makes the decision, she jumps right in with different ideas about how they could spend their time together that would include being more active and cooking healthy meals.

Looking back, I know that my doubts and anxieties took over. Even though I had academic knowledge regarding food justice and healthy food production and consumption as well as personal experience with body image issues, I felt as though it was not my place to share this information with Jestina. There were so many questions looming in my head: What if my recommendations for food choices were beyond her parents' food budget? What if she interpreted my guidance as something she had to do rather than simply advice? Should I be using this as an opportunity to encourage healthy eating or should I really be focusing on helping Jestina accept herself? I do wish I had handled the situation differently. I think as a young person myself without a ton of experience, I got too caught up in my own head and personal issues. In that moment, Jestina needed someone to support her. I do think it is a good idea to think a response through if you have the opportunity to, but I was going overboard. I think previous youth work experience had shaken my confidence and in that moment I felt the repercussions. I wish my initial reaction had been to take a step back and ask why Jestina was feeling this way. I wish I had tried to identify the root cause of the issue. From that, I think an appropriate method of handling the situation would have been far less of a struggle.

Reflection: Kelli realizes that she does have relevant knowledge and experience. However, in the face of the dilemma with Jestina, her knowledge and experience are not actionable. She understands the systems that may constrain Jestina's ability to eat healthily, but she is paralyzed by the enormity of those systems. Rather than being overwhelmed by the questions "looming" in her head, a more experienced youth worker would have asked Jestina more questions to determine the underlying issue and may even have probed about the changes in Jestina's appearance right when they reunited after the summer. Kelli comes to this realization upon reflection, increasing the likelihood that the next time she is in this type of situation, she would approach it differently.

In this dilemma story, Kelli is having a difficult conversation with her long-term mentee in a relatively safe and controlled environment about a struggle that she has gone through in her own life. Kelli's relationship with Jestina allowed her to notice that Jestina was making changes to her appearance. She didn't consider Jestina's changes to be indicative of a problem. However, when Jestina admitted she wanted to be skinnier, Kelli found herself unprepared and unable to respond. Kelli evaluated the issue from multiple perspectives but could not organize her thoughts into a coherent strategy. She jumped from topic to topic in her mind and couldn't identify the angle that would help Jestina the most. Feeling the need to do something, Kelli decided to focus on Jestina's comment directly, without delving into why she raised it. She suggested being active and learning to eat more healthfully. Kelli followed through on this plan with Jestina but did not revisit the topic with her. Upon reflection, Kelli feels she should have asked Jestina more about why she felt that she needed to lose weight rather than getting lost in thinking through every possible angle to the situation. Having had the opportunity to reflect on this dilemma in a structured way, we see great potential for Kelli to improve her practice.

Digging deeper: application to your work

This chapter concludes with three exercises designed to help you develop and refine your ecological intelligence and practice wisdom. We strongly recommend you complete activity one—write your youth worker autobiography—and start activity two—keep a dilemma journal—before reading the remaining chapters in this book.

Activity one: write your youth worker autobiography

Higgs *et al.* claim that professional expertise in human services professions "resides in practice wisdom and practice artistry" (2001: 4). Hildreth and VeLure Roholt (2013) suggest that youth work expertise is connected to the interplay of three forms of knowledge: propositional (formal schooling), practice or professional craft (experience on the job), and personal (life experience). In this first activity, we want you to begin to write your youth work autobiography so that you can explore your "youth work story" and the origins of your practice wisdom and artistry.

- Organize your writing around "critical incidents" that led you to this field and that keep you committed to it. Think intentionally about where your youth work knowledge and skills come from, and include the themes of propositional, professional craft, and personal knowledge in your autobiography.
- Think ecologically about the systems that influenced your development.
- Consider important aspects of your identity such as your age, race, gender, ethnicity, sexual orientation, ability status, and class.
- Consider your history and personal experiences in your family, school, youth development programs, religious institutions, etc.

- Consider the context where you grew up. Was it urban, rural, suburban? In what ways do these dimensions correspond with the youth you work with? How do the similarities and differences present opportunities or challenges in your youth work?

You should think of your autobiography as a work in progress. Your story will deepen the more you reflect on your life experiences, your educational background, and your practice as well as the connections among them. As your story becomes more visible to you, you will be more present in your practice with the youth and will experience new insights into your work.

Activity two: keep a dilemma journal

In order to learn from practice, we recommend that you keep a daily dilemma journal. Every day, jot down some notes about what you struggled with and what you did well. Choose several dilemmas to write about in more depth. Use the following to help guide your journaling:

- Describe the dilemma in as much detail as possible. What was the problem? What were the considerations that needed to be balanced? What did the dilemma make you think about?
- How did the dilemma make you feel? Think about how you felt emotionally as well as how you felt in your body.
- Who were the key actors in the dilemma? Was it a particular youth, a group of youth, a family, a coworker, individuals outside of the program or organization? Describe them in terms of age, gender, race, class, etc. Speculate on what motivated them to act as they did.
- What did you see as the causes of the dilemma, and what did you do to address it?
- How did you decide on that course of action?
- Discuss the outcome of your intervention and evaluate how well you think you handled the dilemma.
- Make a list of all possible other ways to have handled the situation.
- If you were in a similar situation again, would you do the same thing? Why, or why not?

Structured reflection can aid youth workers in establishing a constructive and productive routine of praxis that does not lead to a downward spiral into self-doubt. Journaling can help you discover breakthrough moments in your practice.

Activity three: analyze a dilemma using the Ecological Dilemma Resolution model

Using the EDR model as a lens through which to read youth worker dilemma stories helps us gain insight into how youth workers understand problems of practice and their own decision-making. We see where youth workers get "stuck" in the process of implementing possible solutions. Here is an opportunity to practice using the EDR model.

Below, we share Sylvia's story. As you read it, look for evidence of the two components of the EDR model:

- forms of knowledge required to resolve complex dilemmas of practice; and
- a structured dilemma resolution process.

Reflection questions follow Sylvia's story.

SYLVIA'S STORY

"I don't like you. I don't want you here; you took Maggie's job!" Those were the words that Sasha, a 16-year-old youth leader, flat out told Sylvia during her first few weeks at her new job as Youth/Community Organizer. Having worked in the youth development field for several years, Sylvia was well aware that developing relationships with youth is critical, but after this encounter, she wondered "how do you get teens to trust and confide in you?"

Sylvia grew up in the same city where she now works. She attended high school and college in that city. Her first job working with youth came in her freshman year of high school as a camp counselor. She was amazed that she could get paid to play with kids. After that she knew she wanted to work with youth. Youth work, however, was not an obvious career choice for her. Her family thought she should get a "real job." Under pressure from her family, she spent her first two years in college doing pre-law.

Sylvia persevered, however, and followed her passion. She volunteered as a youth mentor until she got a job as a youth advisor at a college preparatory program. The work was extremely intense. Sylvia found that some of the youth had serious problems with drugs, relationships, and their mental health. She wanted to help them, but as she put it: "I think I put myself out there too much with them. They would call me at 4:00 AM with a crisis and I would be with them all day. ... They had 24/7 access to me. I kind of let them take advantage of me."

The intensity of the situation drove Sylvia to look for a new job. After networking, she found the Youth/Community Organizer position. Several of the youth she mentored previously joined her group at her new organization. But she faced the challenge of developing relationships with the youth already involved in the organization's youth group. She struggled with the question: "How do I get the youth to trust me and confide in me and believe in what I'm doing without necessarily having to be their friend?"

Soon after starting her new job, she began hearing rumors that Iris, one of the young people she was working with, was pregnant and involved in a lot of risky behavior. This young woman had not yet built trust with Sylvia. She wondered: "How do I address that? Do I ask her about it? Is that overstepping some type of boundary?" Sylvia was concerned both with respecting the youth's boundaries and her own, given her prior experience working with young people in crisis. And in the midst of her internal struggle with how to develop relationships and gain trust with the youth who were new to her, Sasha basically told Sylvia she was unwanted and unwelcome. Sasha wouldn't even come upstairs to see her in her office.

Confused by Sasha's powerful reaction, Sylvia asked a few people if they knew where Sasha's anger was coming from. Sylvia found out that Sasha had seen her sitting at Maggie's desk before she had started the job. Apparently Sasha was furious about this. Sylvia recounted Sasha's reaction: "You took over; you're sitting at Maggie's desk. She hadn't even left yet; why were you sitting there?" Apparently, one week, Maggie kind of joked that she was going to leave; and then, two weeks later, she actually did leave. Sylvia reflected:

> Sasha told Maggie a lot of things. There was a day shortly before she left Sasha was talking about her dad being in jail. She was crying, telling her a lot of really personal things. They were really close and then Maggie just left.

Sylvia wanted Sasha to trust her and she wanted to help Iris. She was inclined to connect with them by offering favors of rides and snacks, but she worried about falling into old patterns. Sylvia thought: "I can't let them walk all over me. I just want them to like me and trust me." Sylvia was unsure how to set clear standards with the youth but also be friendly, warm, and accessible enough so that they would come to her if they needed help.

Reflection questions for Sylvia's story

Sylvia grapples with one of the foundational tasks of youth work—forging healthy, trusting relationships with young people. Sylvia's personal struggle with family acceptance of her occupation and her prior challenges establishing healthy boundaries with youth compound the difficulties she faces developing relationships with Sasha and Iris. Her story complicates a typical scholarly reading about the importance of relationships in youth development. Use the following questions to further analyze Sylvia's actions and to think what you would have done if you were in Sylvia's shoes.

1   Describe the characters in this story to the extent that you can. Speculate on what motivates them to act as they do. Are there aspects of Sylvia's identity or background that you think are associated with her approach to developing

relationships with youth? Consider the sources of knowledge that Sylvia is drawing from—personal, propositional, and practice.

2   What would you say are the key challenges in this case? Use the Dilemma Resolution Cycle of problem recognition/appraisal, plan formulation, plan implementation, and evaluation/reflection to understand where Sylvia gets "stuck."

3   Sylvia had a difficult time at a prior organization; how can she develop new ways of thinking about developing relationships with youth at her new organization? What are some things you think Sylvia should do with Sasha and Iris?

Have you ever been in a situation similar to Sylvia's? What have you done to develop relationships with a new group of adolescents?

References

Bessant, J. (2011). Youth work and the education of professional practitioners in Australia. In D. Fusco (Ed.), *Advancing youth work: Current trends, critical questions*. New York: Routledge (pp. 52–68).

Bronfenbrenner, U. (1979). *The ecology of human development: Experiments by nature and design*. Cambridge, MA: Harvard University Press.

Cianciolo, A., Matthew, C., Sternberg, R., and Wagner, R. (2006). Tacit knowledge, practical intelligence, and expertise. In K. A. Ericsson, N. Charness, P. J. Feltovich, and R. R. Hoffman (Eds.), *Cambridge handbook of expertise and expert performance: Its development, organization and content*. Cambridge, UK: Cambridge University Press (pp. 633–52).

Curry, D., Schneider-Munoz, A., Eckles, F., and Stuart, C. (2011). Assessing youth worker competence: National child and youth worker certification. In D. Fusco (Ed.), *Advancing youth work: Current trends, critical questions*. New York: Routledge (pp. 27–38).

Cusick, A. (2001). Personal frames of reference in professional practice. In J. Higgs and A. Titchen (Eds.), *Practice knowledge and expertise in the health professions*. Oxford: Butterworth-Heinemann (pp. 91–5).

Derksen, T. (2010). The influence of ecological theory in child and youth care: A review of the literature. *International Journal of Child, Youth and Family Studies, 1*(3/4), 326–39.

Emslie, M. (2009). Researching reflective practice: A case study of youth work education. *Reflective Practice, 10*(4), 417–27.

Endsley, M. (2006). Expertise and situation awareness. In K. A. Ericsson, N, Charness, P.J. Feltovich, and R. R. Hoffman (Eds.), *Cambridge handbook of expertise and expert performance: Its development, organization and content*. Cambridge, UK: Cambridge University Press (pp. 633–52).

Ericsson, K. A., Charness, N., Feltovich, P. J., and Hoffman, R. R. (Eds.). (2006). *Cambridge handbook of expertise and expert performance: Its development, organization and content*. Cambridge, UK: Cambridge University Press.

Fusco, D. (2012). Use of self in the context of youth work. *Child & Youth Services, 33*(1), 33–45.

Higgs, J. and Bithell, C. (2001). Professional expertise. In J. Higgs and A. Titchen (Eds.), *Practice knowledge and expertise in the health professions*. Oxford: Butterworth-Heinemann (pp. 59–68).

Higgs, J., Titchen, A., and Neville, V. (2001). Professional practice and knowledge. In J. Higgs and A. Titchen (Eds.), *Practice knowledge and expertise in the health professions*. Oxford: Butterworth-Heinemann (pp. 3–9).

Hildreth, R. and VeLure Roholt, R. (2013). Teaching and training civic youth workers: Creating spaces for reciprocal civic and youth development. In R. VeLure Roholt, M. Baizerman, and R. Hildreth (Eds.), *Civic youth work: Co-creating democratic youth spaces*. Chicago: Lyceum Books (pp. 151–9).

Krueger, M. (1997). Using self, story, and intuition to understand child and youth care work. *Child & Youth Care Forum, 26*(3), 153–61.

Larson, R. and Walker, K. (2010). Dilemmas of practice: Challenges to program quality encountered by youth program leaders. *American Journal of Community Psychology, 45*(3–4), 338–49.

Lave, J. and Wenger, E. (1991). *Situated learning: Legitimate peripheral participation*. Cambridge, UK: Cambridge University Press.

Ord, J. (2014). Aristotle's phronesis and youth work: Beyond instrumentality. *Youth and Policy, 112*, 56–73.

Schön, D. (1990). *Educating the reflective practitioner: Toward a new design for teaching and learning in the professions*. San Francisco: Jossey Bass.

Spence, J. (2008). What do you youth workers do? Communicating youth work. *Youth Studies Ireland, 2*(2), 3–18.

Walker, J. and Walker, K. (2011). Establishing expertise in an emerging field. In D. Fusco (Ed.), *Advancing youth work: Current trends, critical questions*. New York: Routledge (pp. 39–51).

Walker, K. and Gran, C. (2010). *Beyond core competencies: Practitioner expertise as a critical component of quality*. St. Paul, MN: University of Minnesota Extension Center for Youth Development.

Walker, K. and Larson, R. (2012). Youth worker reasoning about dilemmas encountered in practice: Expert-novice differences. *Journal of Youth Development, 7*(1), 5–23.

Wood, J., Westwood, S., and Thompson, G. (2015). *Youth work: Preparation for practice*. London: Routledge.

3

NAVIGATING INEXPERIENCE

How reflection guides practice for a novice youth worker

"I was so lost in not knowing what to do."—**Alexandra**

Chapter learning objectives

- Understanding the importance of reflecting with mentors
- Thinking on your feet
- Developing relationships with youth
- Engaging in reflection to advance practice

How can the novice youth worker move beyond the debilitating effects of self-doubt? Walker and Walker (2012) argue that expertise is developed as individuals learn to become deliberate about decisions and judgments. Alexandra, this chapter's youth worker, takes this notion to heart in her trials and tribulations during her first six months as a full-time staff member working at Youth Leadership Academy (YLA), a college access and leadership program for low-income and first-generation college-bound high school students. She began at YLA as a volunteer and quickly moved into a staff position. Alexandra's work at YLA is where her journey towards fostering a deeper understanding of youth development and the complexities of building meaningful relationships with young people began. This chapter explores the development of expertise by a novice youth worker.

As a white, middle-class female who grew up in a small city, Alexandra's childhood was surrounded by diversity on many levels. She was accustomed to being one of the only white people in most of her schools and other settings. However, there was a lot of racial and class segregation in her school, her community, and her neighborhood. While growing up, Alexandra was able to recognize the power and privilege associated with her identity, but she never felt totally comfortable with it. This discomfort drove her to explore issues of social justice in college, which informed her work within youth development and her position at YLA.

Alexandra was hired as the advisor for the sophomore class to replace a staff member who was going on maternity leave. Alexandra was to be responsible for facilitating weekly group meetings with the 15 high school sophomores, meeting individually with each of the students once a month, and co-leading groups and workshops with all of YLA's 60 students. At the same time, Alexandra was beginning to write her master's research paper on the experience of implementing a Social Justice Youth Development (SJYD) curriculum with the sophomore class. Her research required constant and intentional reflection on her work and student reaction. Alexandra approached her work and research with an inward gaze aimed at self-examination that allowed her to track her progress, setbacks, and development.

In this chapter, we see the crippling effects of a novice's self-doubt, the difficulty surrounding how to keep youth at the center of decision-making, and a turnaround towards a transformative approach to youth work. Alexandra makes a deliberate effort to improve her performance through monitoring, planning, reasoning, and anticipating outcomes (Ericsson and Lehmann, 1996; Ericsson et al., 2006). Alexandra's story exemplifies the novice experience as well as the importance of and the need for self-reflection in youth work. As Walker and Walker highlight, "it is not just about going through the motions, but having ongoing opportunities to work at addressing some of the most difficult problems in one's field with coaching, questioning and critical reflection" (2012: 44).

Alexandra's dilemma

Day 1

"Shit, this is real now." My mind could not stop repeating this as I sat in the kitchen at YLA waiting with Rea for the sophomore class to arrive. Rea, the Program Director and former sophomore class advisor at YLA, was about to go on maternity leave and I was taking her place. Shit.

I had spent the last week in August with the sophomores on a camping trip as part of YLA's programming. These trips are set up as a means to foster experiential learning, group cohesion, and familiarity with a non-urban setting. It was a great way to form initial relationships with the youth in the sophomore class; however, it was a very different setting from facilitating group discussions and workshops, which I had never done before. But now my role as advisor was real and I was nervous. Together, Rea and I decided it was best to co-lead the first class meeting in order to more formally discuss the transition of roles and create a smooth transition into the new structure.

My mind raced. How would they perceive me as their new advisor? What if they could tell I was scared? What if they took advantage of my fear? What if I failed? My fear was very present; but also, somewhere, my excitement was too. I had been preparing for this day for the past few months and I knew what I intended to do, say, and expect. So, in some sense, I was ready even though earlier in the day I caught myself fantasizing about "getting sick" so I could call out of work. I was terrified of messing something up without even knowing what exactly that something was. It was like I was attempting to avoid a bad blind date before it even happened by speculating on all the possible negative outcomes. But this was not a blind date; this was my job and although I could not fully trump my fears, I was committed to being present, dedicated, and caring. So the kitchen table is where I sat and waited.

Out of the 15 sophomores, 3 arrived shortly after 2:00, but as time ticked on and the 2:45 starting time grew closer, it was apparent that no one else was going to show up. I knew I should be disappointed, but what I really felt was a sense of relief. The nerves that were crawling within my stomach ceased as I realized that I no longer had to face my fears of leading a group, making a fool of myself, and the students not liking me. So now those fears left me and I relished my newfound ease. But my relief was short-lived, as I realized I would have to deal with the fact that almost no one showed up.

It was clear to me that the sophomores were communicating something that needed to be heard. Was it an act of defiance? A simple, yet bold, message that a new advisor was not an option? Was it a sign about their lack of commitment to the program? Perhaps they hadn't yet felt a sense of accountability to YLA, to each other, and to the advisors? Were there not enough established expectations regarding communication? I wondered how they were supposed to let Rea know if they couldn't make it to a meeting, or if they were supposed to do this at all. Whatever the reason, their ability to control the situation was apparent, and I had to figure out how to effectively begin my role as their new advisor by listening to them while also holding up my own expectations.

Still, I felt very little responsibility for the meeting's low turnout. Since Rea was still around, I assumed it was her duty to make sure students showed up and also to handle the aftermath—which she did, rescheduling the meeting for the next week. I was unsure how to assert my authority and how to embrace my leadership role, so essentially I did not. However, when Rea began her maternity leave a few days after the botched first meeting, I could no longer avoid my doubts and fears. I had to step up and take responsibility.

For the next meeting, I planned to have a discussion about priorities and commitments in order to figure out why people had missed the first meeting. We would then discuss the change in advisors and have time for them to ask me questions, express their concerns, and give feedback about their thoughts for the upcoming year. I wanted to give the class a chance to express themselves and show them that I was there to listen. After, we would reflect on the camping trip with some pictures before starting the first activity called the Power Flower, which would begin my planned curriculum. This was an activity to discuss power and oppression by analyzing how both function in US society and how they are present in our individual social experiences. My idea was to create a space where the sophomores could express their feelings about the changes in the program. I also wanted this to be a space where we could start delving into the topic of social justice so I could start my master's research about facilitating a SJYD curriculum. I was nervous, but I felt prepared. This would soon prove to be a fleeting sensation. Nothing went as planned and another critical challenge emerged as my questions from the week before were answered.

Day 2

As students began to arrive I sat in the kitchen with them. We ate snacks and waited for everyone to come so we could start our meeting at 2:45. During this time, students began to ask me about Rea. They started to tell me that they felt ditched by her, like she didn't care. They questioned me about my role and they talked about some of their dissatisfactions with things like having to choose between sports and YLA, and feeling like individual advising was useless. This onslaught of negative comments surprised me. Even though I had planned to talk about all this in the meeting, I was unsure how to respond. For some reason, I could only envision talking about these issues in the formal group setting, not in the more casual kitchen setting waiting for it to begin. Their honesty and emotion caught me off guard. I knew I was being tested, but I wasn't sure how to get a passing grade with these sophomores.

They were fishing for my thoughts about Rea leaving. They were actively comparing my approach to rules to Rea's and measuring my commitment to them. Driving this were their clear feelings of anger, confusion, and hurt by the loss of Rea and the change to me as their new advisor. They had many questions and I was the person they were looking to for answers, both before the meeting and during it. I was unprepared to answer them and couldn't help but think that Rea was really the person they needed answers from, which would've happened the week before at the originally scheduled first meeting of the year. I was angry with myself for being unprepared and naive, but I projected this anger onto Rea for burdening me with the effects of her lack of effective communication. A part of me knew this was unwarranted, but I was so lost in not knowing what to do that it was the only feeling that I could articulate to myself at the time.

I was forced to think on my feet—something I had very little practice doing in this type of a situation. I told them that Rea wasn't ditching them and that she was having a baby, a reasonable thing to leave work for, but that I could understand how they felt angry and hurt. However, in my head I was flip-flopping. I knew I had to steer the conversation away from them talking badly about my team member, but their disparaging remarks about Rea made me feel like I had an opening to get them to like me. I desperately wanted recognition. I needed this transition to go smoothly. I wanted to be the good guy. Because of my need to be liked and my clouded anger towards YLA and Rea, I don't think I was convincing or strategic enough about how to make clear that she had not ditched them and that she still truly cared.

By the time the formal meeting started, I already doubted myself because I had handled a critical situation poorly. I was questioning my ability to handle tough situations on my feet. Therefore, I made the quick decision to skip my plan to get into why they missed last week and how that reflected on their commitment to YLA. I was nervous about coming across as mean. I wanted to avoid being confrontational and accusatory. So I avoided the topic altogether.

Instead, I asked the students what they wanted to see happen this year at YLA and if they had any questions and concerns for me. This brought up a lot of questions about Rea again, as well as the issue of YLA clashing with other activities and skepticism about my dedication to them as their new advisor. This time, I was stricter about how I handled comments about Rea; I highlighted where I agreed with her about attendance as a crucial component of the program, and I stated that this wasn't the time to criticize her. Additionally, I was honest about my plans for my role at YLA in terms of my position being temporary and having no set plans yet for after graduation. I concluded with saying that I am very committed to being their advisor and that I am open to their feedback all the time. I then moved on, doubtful that my answers were good enough and unsure how to continue responding to them.

I brought out pictures from the camping trip, which got everyone very excited, talkative, and loud. I then asked them to go around and say their favorite part of the trip and what about it they would like to bring back to YLA. Only a few people shared. The other students had side conversations, not paying attention to their fellow students. Some just got up and left the room. A few times I asked people to be quiet, but I didn't want to constantly be reprimanding them so I didn't address every instance of what I perceived as disrespect. I couldn't just yell, "shut up!" even though those two words were going through my head. I didn't want to create that kind of authoritative environment I knew they must experience at school, but I also didn't want an environment where I couldn't maintain respect and control of the class. I had no idea what I was doing and I felt my inadequacy creeping all around me. But I kept going on with the day, squirming in my self-doubt.

I proceeded to introduce the Power Flower, an activity that analyzed power and privilege from a societal and then individual level. As a whole, we filled out the flower's outer petal with the social groups that have power in American society. This went well. People were relatively engaged and interested, and some people expressed how they liked having an interactive meeting. At the same time, however, there were comments about how they always talk about racism, sexism, and inequality at YLA and how it can be tiring. I could sense that I was losing their attention and intrigue as people started having side conversations and were leaving the room. Still, I continued.

They then individually filled in the inner petals with their own identities and counted how many matched the outer petals in order to see where they did and didn't fall into the power groups identified earlier. Before we got to discuss the activity and reflect on its meaning, three students announced that they had to leave for their volleyball game. Another left shortly after because her ride had arrived. Once they left, the others became disengaged. I attempted to regain attention and have a discussion about the point of the activity. I managed to get one student to answer. He said, "to make us feel bad." This was the kind of response I was expecting and I told him my intention wasn't that but, rather, to acknowledge the realities of our society and how there are systems that create barriers for certain people. I then urged him to elaborate, but he didn't. Instead, he said that he scored an 11 and asked if there was anyone that scored higher. I told him I got a 12. He then said, "Ohhh, it's because you can put that you're white." I said, "I know, so what does that mean?" No one responded or seemed interested. Instead they were getting ready to leave or talking to each other; some were even listening to music. I kept going and talked about my interpretation of what the purpose of the activity was, and how just because I am white and their advisor does not mean that I have to necessarily have all the power in this meeting space and beyond, and that hopefully we can work to change that. However, I had lost complete control at this point and it was clear that the meeting was over even though it was before the scheduled 4:45 end time.

When the meeting had ended and everyone left, I reflected on it through writing and with some discussion with my coworker Marc. I was disappointed with myself for being unable to control the meeting better, confused at my lack of preparation regarding the students' reaction to losing Rea, and angry at my overall naiveté. I questioned my abilities as a youth worker, wondered how I could make the class interested and engaged, and thought about ways to create firm rules about attendance. However, the most fundamental question I had to ask myself was whether or not I should continue with the curriculum I had produced. The students' comments about their dislike of talking all the time about racism, sexism, and inequality could not be overlooked, and their unwillingness to complete the Power Flower activity stuck with me. While I was aware that this reaction could be attributed to internalized oppression and could give me an opportunity to prove the relevance of social justice issues, there were clearly other issues at play that could also have led to their disinterest. Additionally, I began to realize that I had no idea how to deliver social justice ideals to young people, especially as a white woman with youth of color. I wondered whether it was really fair of me to still be learning about the SJYD framework and attempting to understand my own social identity while at the same time administering a curriculum aimed at having youth do the exact same thing?

I quickly began to view the curriculum as too constraining. It gave me too many unrealistic expectations about the students' responses and outcomes because it was clear, for various reasons, that the class was not yet at a point where these types of discussions would be accepted and I was also not in a place where I was completely comfortable being the one to facilitate them. Through talking with Marc and via my own reflections, I decided to put aside the outline of my curriculum and, instead, to work on building group identity and morale in the class meetings while also creating meaningful relationships with each student through individual advising once a month. I wanted to discover what the class was interested in and passionate about so that they could have more ownership over their time at YLA. This meant generating meeting topics and goals on a week-to-week basis so that I could take into account what had gone on during previous class meetings, community meetings, and individual advising. It felt like a more personalized approach to what the class needed; however, my research was still looming over my head and I could not neglect the data I planned to collect regarding the students' growth in terms of SJYD.

The first four months

What followed was a series of class meetings during November and December that covered topics such as: the importance of being part of a group and the inherent potential for power that this collectivity brings; democracy and economic inequality in relation to the Occupy Movement that had been active at the time; and community mapping in order to generate consensus on an issue to get involved with in the greater community. I wanted to encourage the class to see themselves as a group, and I challenged them to do something together.

I perceived that these meetings were, on the whole, received well by the sophomores as they seemed more intrigued and engaged. However, they were also riddled with dilemmas I was facing surrounding discipline, the students' ability to listen to and respect one another and myself, and how to keep the class focused. They were often a rowdy group, and while this made for lots of excitement and energy, it also created chaos and divergences from topic discussions which were hard for me to handle. All the while, I was meeting with the sophomores one-on-one, learning more about them as individuals and sharing parts of myself as well.

During these few months, I was feeling very up and down about my role at YLA as an advisor. I constantly doubted myself and felt isolated as a new staff member. I was unsure what kind of impact, if any at all, I was having on the sophomores, and I felt as though the class meetings were boring and meaningless. I was also worried that my research would fail because I was having trouble getting parental consent forms back in order to record the meetings. I also questioned my ability and effectiveness in terms of delivering a social justice-oriented program. I wanted more guidance and was bad at asking for help; but when I did, the conversations I had with Marc were very influential. He made suggestions that made me see situations differently and consider new aspects of specific incidences, and showed me that discussion and reflection with team members are vital to a program's success.

After a particularly chaotic meeting, I asked for Marc's support. I expressed not only my worry that I could not control the group well enough in terms of their behavior and interest level, but also that I felt unable to effectively and thoroughly explain the meaning behind the activities I presented to the class. While both of these had to do with my lack of confidence, Marc made me realize that they also have to do with issues surrounding listening and communication, and being able to think on my feet when I see a teachable moment. So he suggested that I do some sort of listening activity at my next class meeting. I liked this idea and found a way to do it where I could incorporate three very important topics that bridged together many of the goals I had for the year: listening and responding to each other constructively; learning about each other in order to develop trust and a positive group dynamic; and self-discovery through reflecting on personal identity. Not only did the next meeting in the middle of January take me by surprise but it was also an incredible and critical turning point for me as an advisor, the growth of the class, and the direction of my research.

The turning point

I began the meeting by introducing the opening activity as a listening exercise. I told them I was going to read them an essay I had written during my freshman year at college about the history of my education and that I just wanted them to listen and respond with any questions or comments after I finished. Some students asked if they could get more comfortable and turn off the lights, which I thought was fine. So we all sat in a circle with the lights off, and although it might have felt a bit like elementary school story time, this actually set the mood that was essential to the flow of the meeting.

I was nervous. I have never liked sharing personal information about myself to anyone, let alone a group of people. But I shared my essay anyway. It told of my journey through bilingual education, my experience in school being white among my Latino peers, my struggle to comprehend white privilege, and my later toils with feeling uninterested and unprepared for college. I expressed many personal details of my life and revealed transitional points where I came to pivotal realizations about my identity and my values. There were times when my voice shook a bit and my nervousness was visible, but when I finished, the class applauded and responded by saying they liked it and commenting that they felt surprised to learn so much about me and past things I've struggled with. I was glad because I wanted them to learn more about me, and I talked about the importance of storytelling as a source of communication and discovery.

I then challenged each of them to share their story with the group at some point throughout the year. This brought up some confusion about what I meant by "their story." So I asked: "If someone were to ask you, 'what's your story?', how would you respond? What events and experiences have shaped who you are?" They seemed to understand this better, so I asked if anyone wanted to share right then. There was silence and some nervous laughter, and initially I assumed no one would, which was fine since I had a plan for the rest of the meeting. I waited as we all looked from one person to the next. Thinking I might have to move on, I asked one last time if anyone else wanted to share and said that I'd ask next meeting as well. I waited a bit and, as I was about to start the next activity, the student to my right, Ronnie, spoke up and said he wanted to share his story. We all sat back and gave him our attention. He told a story of his alcoholic and abusive father and his family's move from Florida to escape him; how Ronnie's grandparents rejected him and his siblings for being biracial; and his self-discovery and acceptance of being gay. His poise, maturity, and honesty were impressive. He inspired all of his fellow students to share their stories that day as well.

They spoke of parents getting divorced, moving from house to house and from state to state, near death experiences, coming to the US, feeling excluded in middle school, pushing for gender equality in church, abuse, financial struggles, attempts to fit in, and more. Some cried and were comforted, others made the group laugh, and everyone was heard. Everyone was unraveled as they revealed the complexities of their lives. It was apparent that each student wanted to be heard and to be known by the group, but it also seemed as though they felt somewhat accountable to each other to share their stories. I was there to respond and lead the meeting, but the students dictated its flow and shaped the space into one where everyone felt comfortable and safe. The meeting ended with one student suggesting that we have a group hug. We all embraced and laughed, and I couldn't have felt more proud.

Throughout and after the meeting, I was completely floored. I had not expected it to be so powerful and personal, and I was impressed by what the sophomores had accomplished. It was moving and incredibly meaningful for everyone involved, and it had created a starting point for the class to grow together. I wrote in my journal: "This was the first meeting where I came away with more positive feelings than negative ones. I am very hopeful." For the first time, I did not immediately doubt myself but, instead, felt truly confident. I felt like I had done something right and impactful, which made me look forward to future meetings instead of worrying about how to avoid whatever mistakes I believed I would inevitably make at the next one. It was as though this newfound energy gave the class and me the ability to tackle any difficult topic or task; it was clear that the sophomores and I were finally on the same page. This meeting created a space for each student to begin the process of self-awareness—the phase of my curriculum that I had skipped over but which was now clearly needed. I knew where to begin anew.

I decided that the rest of the year would focus on self-awareness and identity development. I realized that this could be a longer process than anticipated, and while I would be going back to my original curriculum, I didn't want to limit myself to a strict set of activities and topics to cover. So we had meetings where we discussed topics ranging from gender in the media to analysis of stereotypes to racial inequality. We attended a rally for Trayvon Martin and another one to raise awareness for equal access to education for immigrant students. However, we also covered topics where the students designed their ideal YLA, practiced interviewing for jobs, performed skits, and at times just played games. I was now more aware that unexpected occurrences could and would dictate a meeting, which wasn't necessarily a negative thing. This allowed the meetings to feel more organic because the flow developed mostly from the students; I just had to figure out how to facilitate what they created. Additionally, I even found that I worked better without a specific outline for the meeting's agenda. I was getting better at thinking on my feet, creating and confronting conflict, and shaping the meetings by responding to what I perceived the sophomores needed as the year went by. I was more confident, less rigid, and considering more with every meeting and encounter

I had with the class. I realized that while still quite challenging and riddled with dilemmas, I was actually enjoying my job.

Unpacking the dilemma

> We need to overcome self-limiting beliefs and practices that hold us back from reaching our potential
> —Ingrid Chapman (anti-racist organizer) in Crass (2013: 274)

This dilemma provides us with a painfully familiar glimpse into beginners' experiences of stumbling over both youth and themselves before getting the hang of good practice. While it is normal for novice youth workers to experience anxiety about how to work with youth and achieve program outcomes, Alexandra's struggles are exacerbated by the pressure of working within a Social Justice Youth Development (SJYD) model committed to maintaining an anti-oppressive and anti-authoritarian stance. The tension of educating youth about power and oppression but not creating an atmosphere of indoctrination or "power over" is nuanced and difficult for even the most experienced SJYD workers. For Alexandra, reflection was at first paralyzing as she overanalyzed her failures and tended to ignore success or insights about her daily practice. But later, when she sought out help from a mentor, she grew more confident in her practice, was able to become more flexible with her program, and started to actually enjoy the work. We now use the Ecological Dilemma Resolution model to analyze Alexandra's case.

Knowledge

Alexandra comes to youth work without a great deal of personal or practice-based experience. She acknowledges that although she grew up in a diverse community and that she was aware of her privilege, she never fully explored it or made meaning of it before college. In college, she chose to study power and oppression by majoring in Sociology and concentrating on Youth Studies. It was propositional knowledge that fueled Alexandra's desire to work with young people in a SJYD framework rather than prior life or professional experience.

In SJYD programming, issues of power and oppression are focused upon as lessons that can aid youth in navigating their daily lives and community. SJYD programs seek to reflect this mission by striving for egalitarian relationships between youth and adults. This magnified importance of power inequity can lead to hypersensitivity for adult youth workers, which prevents them from feeling at ease in their role. We see this when Alexandra begins to doubt her ability to work through a social justice lens because she is a white college-educated woman and her youth are largely low-income youth of color. This fear of replicating oppressive power dynamics through "white saviorism," adultism, or other forms of inequalities can lead to a lack of action and discipline in order to remain uncontrolling and anti-authoritarian, or to avoid the pretension of explaining oppression to those that live with it daily.

Dilemma Resolution Cycle

Initially, rather than using the Dilemma Resolution Cycle to advance her practice, Alexandra appears to go around and around the cycle without gaining many insights into how to improve her practice. She identifies problems, decides what she is going to do about them, half-heartedly implements her plans, and then reflects that she is failing at youth work. If we look closer at each step of the process, we can understand more specifically where she gets stuck. For purposes of this analysis, we will focus on her initial encounter with the youth that first afternoon in YLA's kitchen.

Problem identification

She goes into her first encounter with the youth feeling intellectually but not emotionally prepared. She has her curriculum; she has her opening speech. But she is also full of dread and worry. And then the youth don't show up! And she is relieved! Relieved until she realizes this is now her problem to address. She has an analysis of why they did not come. In her analysis of the problem, she concludes that the youth are testing her, that they are expressing their dissatisfaction with the program, and that they are communicating their sadness about losing Rea.

Plan formulation

She realizes that she is faced with a complex dilemma. She has to be there for the youth and help them through their sense of loss, and she has to establish herself as the new advisor. Her plan involves using the next meeting to process Rea's leaving, to explore the level of the youth's commitment to YLA, and to establish her expectations for the group.

Plan implementation

This is where Alexandra gets stuck. She is unable to implement the plan she devises. The next week, she waits in the kitchen again for the youth to come. This time they arrive and they are full of questions and opinions. The session was not going as she anticipated! The youth were pushing her for information in the informal space of the kitchen rather than in the meeting that she had planned. Instead of using the kitchen encounter to meet the youth where they are, she panics. She engages in conversation, all the while ruminating that if they would just wait for the meeting then she would have all the answers for them there! She doesn't fully engage in the kitchen, and then, because she has been thrown off her game by the kitchen interaction, she decides to scratch the whole conversation about group commitments in the official meeting. Instead she moves directly into her curriculum.

Evaluation/reflection

Alexandra focuses her reflection on her inability to think on her feet. She realizes that the kitchen conversation would have been an excellent opportunity to engage with the youth, but she becomes aware that she doesn't know how to be flexible and seize the teachable moment. She also realizes she avoided the difficult conversation with the youth because of her need to be liked by them and for them not to think she was mean. While these reflections are insightful, she largely beats herself up for her inability to think on her feet and does not push herself to learn from this moment. She works from a position of self-doubt for several months.

We see Alexandra repeating this debilitating cycle over and over during her first several months. She sticks to lesson plans because they keep her grounded even though she realizes she isn't reaching the youth, but she holds on to her plans because she has trouble thinking on her feet. Over time, she comes to understand that youth work is about creating a more youth-centered space, based on mutual respect and the fluid needs of youth rather than the rituals of a planned curriculum. She begins to realize that a youth worker's day may be planned beforehand, but she/he should be ready to fall into a new groove or mesh her/his plans with the dilemmas of the day. Alexandra, early on, had created a narrow curriculum and plan for youth. While a plan is important, knowledge that this plan must be flexible and change in relation to youth directions emerged through a learning curve. Alexandra eventually learns that to authentically teach material on social justice issues, one must become vulnerable in order to build trust and establish relationships with youth.

When Alexandra is finally able to shift her analysis of the problem away from her own shortcomings and toward figuring out what the youth need, she is able to unlearn some bad habits and realize more fully a *relationship* with the young people. Marc's mentorship proved to be critically important in her ability to make this shift. Originally Alexandra creates a curriculum in which youth are meant to listen to her, but Marc encourages her to listen to the youth. She opens herself up to the youth and becomes vulnerable with them. Youth work finally becomes a mutual experience in which the lived experience of young people becomes a body of knowledge and her training and skill sets are a tool for collective transformation.

REFLECTING ON PRACTICE:

What does Alexandra do well in this story? What strengths does she bring to youth work?

Where does Alexandra get stuck in this story? What keeps her from moving through the Dilemma Resolution Cycle?

What advice would you have given Alexandra if you were her mentor?

In what ways can you relate to Alexandra's experience? Have you ever had the kind of feelings of self-doubt and paralysis she expresses? What helped you push through?

Summary

Reflection is critical to good youth work, yet in Alexandra's case, it tended to be more paralyzing than cathartic. Part of what makes Alexandra's self-reflection such a stumbling block is that it is focused more on her own failings than it is in creating a new direction or solution. Repeatedly focusing on the bad prevented Alexandra from seeing the good and expanding it. Praxis cycles from self-reflection and constructive criticism into a renewed plan for action. Alexandra perhaps became more bogged down in the preoccupation of self-critique than in rejuvenation. This eventually changes as Alexandra becomes more comfortable with the idea of working with youth, as she builds trust and respect with youth, and as she works in a positive direction alongside her coworker and mentor, Marc.

While self-awareness is useful (and necessary), fear is not useful. Social justice organizers need to learn that leadership and teaching, even as people with privilege, is important. Stepping back from addressing these issues because it is power laden isn't really a solution to that inequality. What is important is that privileged adults remain aware and reflective of their power, but use this in ways that empower others. Mistakes of course will be made! It's not about making no mistakes; it's about moving. As Martin Luther King said: "If you can't fly, run. If you can't run, walk. If you can't walk, crawl. But by all means, keep moving." The courage to make those mistakes on a path toward collective liberation is more valued than the fear to move at all. To remain humble and accepting of youth perspectives and discussions on oppression is important in building a process of mutual learning and trust around the subject.

From Alexandra's dilemma, we gain insights into lessons for novice youth workers. The crucial aspects of reflection and praxis, the usefulness of mentoring with more experienced youth workers, and the building up of trust and respect between adults and young people before tackling hard personal topics are the big three. Maintain confidence when working with youth, humility and equity when discussing social justice issues, and the flexibility of planning to make sure that the daily tumble does not unhinge high standards for youth.

The anti-racist feminist organizer Chris Crass outlines a praxis-based set of questions that may aid youth workers in a "focus on assets rather than deficits" (2013: 276):

- What went well?
- What am I (or we) good at?
- What are the things I take for granted about this situation, organization, experience that I actually really appreciate?
- What are the positives that can help us achieve our goals, improve our weaknesses, and give us momentum to move forward?
- How have we taken on challenges and improved in the past, and what can we learn from that to help us continue to do that now and tomorrow?
- What did I accomplish today?

Digging deeper: applying the dilemma to your work

Activity 1: reflecting with mentors

Identify a coworker at your organization, or at a similar youth-serving agency, with whom you can reflect on your practice. Take a recent issue where you felt stuck or like you had little control. Bring this issue to this coworker/mentor. Get their opinion. Do role plays with them to practice possible solutions and model potential youth reactions to these tactics.

Activity 2: one-to-ones (part one)

Make a plan to do one-to-ones with the youth you work with. One-to-ones with youth can help novice youth workers build a sense of trust with youth. One-to-ones can help a SJYD youth worker to build relationships with youth before they begin talking about potentially painful subjects that link the political with the personal. Pick one youth in your organization you will get to know on a personal level this week. Ask them about "their story": What is their family life like? Who raised them and where? What do they struggle with? What are their passions and dreams? The following week, pick another young person and continue the process. Be prepared to share your story with the youth.

Activity 3: where do you get stuck?

Identify areas where you feel like you get stuck as a youth worker. Is it managing large groups, dealing with defiance, or talking about race or sexuality? Make a list of the topics or situations you know that you struggle with. What is it about these that make you uncomfortable? For each sticky situation, decide on three things you can do to increase your comfort level with it. Ask peers how they deal with these particular situations.

Activity 4: think on your feet! (part one)

Increase you mental flexibility by running through "what if" situations. You can do this alone or with a group. Write down possible trip-ups in your plans/curriculum and play them out. Come up with a plan B for all your plans (e.g. your plan is to do role plays on communication with youth and no one will get up to act theirs out). Remember to relax; don't put so much pressure on yourself to get everything *right*. Our goal is growth, not perfection. Never forget that youth development is a long process of mutual growth; it cannot be completed or ruined in a day.

References

Crass, C. (2013). *Towards collective liberation: Anti-racist organizing, feminist praxis, and movement building strategy*. Oakland, CA: PM Press.

Ericsson, K. A. and Lehmann, A. C. (1996). Expert and exceptional performance: Evidence of maximal adaptation to task constraints. *Annual Review of Psychology, 47,* 273–305.

Ericsson, K. A., Charness, N., Feltovich, P. J., and Hoffman, R. R. (Eds.). (2006). *Cambridge handbook of expertise and expert performance: Its development, organization and content.* Cambridge, UK: Cambridge University Press.

Walker, J. and Walker, K. (2012). Establishing expertise in an emerging field. In D. Fusco (Ed.), *Advancing youth work: Current trends, critical questions.* New York: Routledge (pp. 39–51).

4

BALANCING HIGH EXPECTATIONS, PROGRAM STRUCTURE, AND YOUTH REALITIES

Making kids fit the program or the program fit the kids

Chapter learning objectives

- Recognizing when personal triggers or disappointments in youth performance cloud judgment
- Knowing when to be flexible with program rules and standards to ensure youth can benefit from the program
- Navigating conflicting expectations among home, school, and a youth program

Youth work creates spaces in which young people can develop their interests, abilities, and skills. Due to the relational nature of the work, youth workers learn about young people's goals. They become the person who alternately reminds youth about their goals and provides support so that they can achieve them. Youth with challenging backgrounds or who lack family support need this type of inspiration and structure most of all, yet can oftentimes have a hard time complying with program guidelines and expectations. Youth workers have to learn to strike an ever-changing balance among three dynamics: 1) maintaining high standards for all youth, 2) providing support and structure to ensure youth can meet these expectations, and 3) tailoring the program or the expectations for youth whose individual situations, complex histories, and unique needs may prevent them from "fitting" into a given structure or from being able to achieve program standards.

This chapter explores the stories of two youth workers—Melinda and Loren—who struggle to include youth who would benefit most but who are not complying with the expectations of the program. Melinda works in the city where she grew up. She runs an award-winning dance team at a local youth organization. Loren grew up in a small suburb about 50 miles from the city where she now works as an instructor in a high school diploma equivalency (GED) program at a drop-in youth center.

Melinda, as a community insider, and Loren, as an outsider, reflect on their decisions to be too hard or too soft on the youth and the results of these decisions. Both youth workers have to choose whether they should change program expectations for particular youth, push those youth harder to adhere to a uniform set of guidelines, or ask those young people to leave the programs. They struggle so intensely because both have the interests of the youth at the center of their analysis; however, knowing what to do to support these youth is not clear. These stories demonstrate just how challenging it is for youth workers to achieve the right balance that ensures maximum participation and maximum benefit—both over the short term and the long term. In spite of their different positions and backgrounds, they come to a similar conclusion in their dilemma resolution process.

Introducing Melinda

> *"I know that the real world will make no exceptions or excuses for them."*— **Melinda**

Melinda got into youth work through a high school job at an after-school youth program. She had gone to that program as a child and remembered having a really good time there. Later, as an employee, she felt it was one of the best, most rewarding jobs she ever had because she felt that they were really affecting the youth. She was able to integrate her passion for the arts into her job by running music groups and a choir, and by directing shows. When Melinda went to college, she participated in three different dance teams and built her artistic skills, while maintaining her love for youth work. She now runs Synergy—an award-winning dance team organized through the local Boys and Girls Club—where her energy, dedication, and no-nonsense attitude carries over. Her role as dance coach involves much more than teaching steps though; on a typical day, she spends her time planning the schedule, buying supplies for activities, doing paperwork, dealing with parent concerns, planning fundraisers, and making plans to improve her program for the next year. This all gets done in the hour before her program or on her own time the night before. It's a hectic schedule to keep the team going, but she feels that the lessons the youth learn there are important and can really help to prepare the youth for a future where they can succeed.

Melinda's dilemma

Technically my job is to teach dance. But it's more than that. The dancing is just what gets them in the room. I see that my main job is to teach the youth about respect, accountability, and character building. I don't just want to teach them about these ideas, but how to live them. I hold them accountable and make them take responsibility for their actions. If I see they have an issue with somebody, I'll say: "If you have an issue with somebody and it bothers you that bad, you take them to the side and you talk about it. If you can't do that, then there's no issue, right? Why are you talking behind their back?" I don't let things pass and they know it. If I hear them talking about something that's going on in the streets, I come to them and I call them on it. They know what I expect of them. I hold them accountable and I make them hold each other accountable for what they say and what they do. Sometimes I see them hanging out with their boyfriend, not doing their homework, and I'll call them out like, "do you know that your girlfriend does no work?" and they're like, "aw come on!" I don't care; everybody needs to know. They should be embarrassed. I'll even call them out when grades come in, telling everyone to come look.

I try to explain to them that everything we learn in dance goes to every part of your life. I say:

> If you know you have dance every Tuesday at 4:00 then why are you telling me you need to skip practice to do homework? Why didn't you take care of that before practice? These are the things that you're going to encounter when you go to college or when you go to a job. I know I go to work every Monday so, unless it's something really important, why am I trying to paint my toes, right, when I'm supposed to be at work?

I try to teach them those things and I'm honest with them; there are things that I mess up—we all mess up sometimes—but you need to know the expectations and deal with the consequences if you don't meet those expectations.

But this work is hard—this deeper life work. Sometimes I wonder why it seems like I care more about these kids' future than they do. I remember one of my girls was just telling me about her plan to go to California to "make it" after high school. I just told her straight up:

> Don't tell people you're going to California; you're not going anywhere. What are you doing now to get to California tomorrow? Nothing. I see you in the hallway when everyone else is doing their homework, and you're going to California?—maybe in your head.

I really struggle with this. How do I motivate girls like this? I want to push them, to tell them they can do so much more. But I also don't want to push so hard or expect so much that they can never achieve what I'm asking. I also wonder if it's possible to have the same expectations for all my kids, or if I should make exceptions for some of their life circumstances. I'm conflicted because I want to help build them up, but I also know that the real world will make no exceptions or excuses for them.

It's hard though, and sometimes I feel like giving up because it can be so challenging to try and get these kids to see more for themselves. But I don't because I just feel like they're not hearing this stuff from anybody else. For some kids, the culture that they live in at home is the culture that I'm trying to have them fight against. It's discouraging for me. For example, I asked one of my dancers about her report card. We talked about her grades. The next day I asked her what her mom said about her report card. She said, "My mom never asked me for my report card." That was so discouraging. I start to wonder why I'm trying so hard if I'm the only one who cares about their future. But I know I can't give up.

Right now, I have 40 kids on the dance team. Most are doing well in school and a few are in high honors and take a lot of Advanced Placement (AP) classes, but I have three that are basically flunking. My rule is that you're not supposed to dance if you're not making your grades. But I keep those three on to watch them. One of the girls who is failing is Vanessa. She is in the seventh grade and she has already stayed back once. She had danced when she was younger, but when she got into middle school, she started to withdraw. She became what we call a "hallway kid"—one of the kids who roam the hallways because they aren't in any of the activities. Because of my past relationship with her, I took a chance and brought her onto the team.

Her aunt tells me there has been an improvement in her motivation and attitude since she joined the team; however, her schoolwork has remained problematic. It looks like she's going to have to repeat the seventh grade again. Now what do I do? Do I kick her off the team or suspend her because she's not making her grades? Will kicking her off put her at risk of backsliding even more? Do I make an exception for her and keep her on the team? But what kind of message does that send to the other kids, or even to her? So far, the other girls have not said anything about me breaking my own rule. I think it's because of the lessons I taught them. They don't say anything about the kids who are failing staying on the team. Some kids will even say things like, "She needs this so I don't think you should just let her go." I have others that will help the other girls with their homework and writing papers.

Even though the other kids are okay with them staying on the team, I'm torn. There are a limited number of slots on the team and it's pretty competitive. We have no money and we have to do a lot of fundraising on our own. The size of the team is limited by how many I can fit on our bus because I can't afford to transport any more girls. Aside from the cost factor, I believe it is so important to hold the kids to a high standard, especially because no one else in their lives does. But what am I risking if I keep my tougher kids who don't meet the expectations out of the shows, or even cut them from the team? I'm afraid that if I exclude Vanessa then it will jeopardize some of the improvements we've seen in her behavior and attitude. But if I keep her, I'm afraid the kids will think they can get over on stuff and take advantage of the fact that I have too much heart. When they leave the Club, the world won't give them so many breaks. Next year, I will be stricter on the grades from the beginning. I'm just going to have to figure out a way to be tougher. I think if I can have them from the beginning, they will live up to the expectation. They just have to do better. I tell them all the time, "You have to do more for yourself." And that's the truth.

Introducing Loren

"I know that these students don't need another hard lesson. They've experienced so many in their relatively short lifetime. What they need is a chance."—**Loren**

Loren is the sole instructor for a high school equivalency (GED) program located at a drop-in youth center. The center serves young people aged 14–24. Its members receive free educational, health, work readiness, and leadership opportunities. Although any youth within the age range can be a member, many of the structured programs target particular youth. The bilingual English/Spanish GED program admits students aged 16–24 who have not earned a high school diploma and are not engaged in a traditional school.

Loren finds it ironic that she is even in a position as a teacher because of her ambivalent attitude toward academia and formal education. She is grateful for her college experience and stuck with the classes because she did see the value in the diploma. But her real learning happened in what she calls "the trenches," outside the formal classroom, in the community.

She encourages her students to get their GED even though she doesn't necessarily believe that the things they learn in the classroom are the most important to know. But she knows the diploma will open doors for them so she encourages her students to stick with it. Loren's fundamental goal in this program is to advance students' grade levels and ultimately produce GED graduates. But she has bigger goals than that. She wants her students to love learning. She wants to set them on a course to becoming lifelong learners. This is very challenging given her students' backgrounds and negative experiences with formal schooling; but she had been successful with both goals over the years. Loren's dilemma is about a group of students who, due to their particularly difficult classroom behaviors, made her question whether she could even stay at her job.

Loren's dilemma

CARL: "What's on your face? Are those pimples?" (directed at Loren during class)
JULIE: "That's mad disrespectful. You are so inappropriate."
CARL: "Well, you're mad disrespectful and inappropriate."
DENNIS: "But really, what is that on your face?"

This exchange among an 18-year-old and two 19-year-olds was typical during our GED classes. I would be trying to work with students as a group and individually on their lessons, and this trio would disrupt class with irrelevant, often negative arguments, remarks, and interactions. Externally, I would roll with the punches and use as many tricks as possible to redirect each individual back to his/her work. But day after day it grew to be a seemingly impossible challenge since all three of these students craved the spotlight and knew how to insert themselves into a moment for attention.

As time went on, I knew I had to deal with these students' disruptive behaviors. So in early spring, I met individually with each student that I felt was detracting from the classroom culture of learning and respect. I invited our on-site mental health counselor to join these conversations. In these meetings, we discussed how the student could adhere to classroom expectations. I developed an agreement with each student who met with me and essentially suspended/expelled by default those who were unwilling to sit with me and the counselor. I think most students felt targeted and demonized by these meetings because they were not ready to change and therefore, one by one, they stopped coming to class. So while I felt uncomfortable with this approach and was not proud that these students left, I was relieved that their incessant disruptive behavior would no longer interrupt the learning of the other students.

Then in early September, one by one, they started to drop by the Center again; Carl, Julie, and Dennis. After a six-month hiatus, these young people were asking to return to class. Normally I am thrilled when students decide to give the GED program another try. I intentionally run a very flexible program knowing that our students come from tough backgrounds and have had bad experiences in traditional school environments. I try to meet young people where they are at, rather than forcing arbitrary attendance rules and standards on them. Most of my students need flexibility, support, and understanding in order to successfully pass the test. I have seen even the most disengaged students complete their GED when they decide they are ready to take the next steps in their lives.

But this group of students? Just the idea that they were coming back made me dread my job. I immediately felt triggered. All of my senses were exaggerated and distorted. Individually, I knew each of these students needed extra support due to a myriad of circumstances; together they created a stressful, seemingly impossible situation for me. I told the Director that "if this group reforms, I won't like my job anymore." I have managed difficult group dynamics before, but this was over the top! Something about the group dynamic and some students in particular made me feel especially uncomfortable, and I surely didn't have control of the situation. The students were running the show and I was half present and half in another world.

As each of these students started approaching me to return to class, I considered my old strategy to either isolate them into their own separate space or to exclude them altogether. These students had been MIA for months and part of me wanted to punish them for not showing up, for not taking the class seriously. The power was all mine; I didn't have to take them back. I knew I could make them learn the hard way but this did not feel right. I felt like my decision would have so many effects in the future. I asked myself "why would you not take them?" And all I could come up with was to teach them a lesson. That just didn't sit right with me.

I've heard the saying from many, including youth workers, that "you can't let one bad apple spoil the bunch" when questions about kicking misbehaving youth come up. But I didn't feel like that solution produced a long-term resolution. I knew at some level I felt uncomfortable when Julie, Dennis, and Carl left the last time. These students have what I consider to be great challenges in their life. Carl continually was dealing with housing challenges and was always on the verge of homelessness; Dennis was involved with a gang and the drama followed him wherever he went; and Julie had a new boyfriend and was therefore kicked out of her mother's house. I realized that I must have been in a triggered space because I knew that these students didn't need another hard lesson; they'd experienced so many in their relatively short lifetime. What they needed was a chance.

I shifted to a more compassionate perspective, asking myself questions such as: "Isn't it my job to handle any type of situation, to meet young people where they're at, and to teach all youth who say they want to take part?" I also thought about the effects on the program's reputation. How do I maintain the culture of learning and respect while still accepting all who apply to my program?

The solution I came up with, after much brainstorming and sitting with ideas, was to break the student body into three classes, each meeting for 4.5 hours per week instead of the 12–14-hour weeks I was offering. I decided to go for quality over quantity. I realized that many students, most in fact, did not take advantage of the 12–14 hours per week of class time, so I let go of the guilt about reducing the hours. Furthermore, and more importantly, I shifted my response from reactionary to proactive; I made the change my choice and my desire, not any student's fault.

In determining the students for each of the three classes, I thoroughly analyzed each student individually and in relation to every other student. I consulted with other staff and reviewed the attendance patterns of each student. I came up with a list that I then sat with for almost a week, changing a name here and there along the way. I also started announcing a change in the schedule to students, one by one, waiting to see what kind of response I would get. No one seemed too upset. I kept moving slowly with my plan.

Finally in late September, I composed a letter in English and Spanish that announced the change. I wrote that I was overwhelmed with the number of students all at once; I needed to come up with a different plan. I owned the need for change and the problem. I told students that I wanted to give more focused time to each and every one of them and, as it was, I couldn't do that. I gave each her/his days and time of class and encouraged them to come on time and take full advantage of me in a small class setting. I had three people proofread my letter to make sure it was just right; I was nervous about delivering it and wanted to make sure my message was clear and concise.

Those who received the letter on the first day seemed a bit shocked. The students were comparing schedules; some were quiet and others were vocally upset. I reiterated to anyone that wanted to discuss the changes in the program that I was open to that, but that this was something I had to do to be able to do my job well and that I thought it would give more individual time for each of them. That particular explanation seemed to satisfy the complaints.

I received a handful of very positive, affirming responses as well. One student who had worked with me two years earlier and had recently returned said: "Wow, I wanted this when I was here before. It took you this long to figure it out?!" A few other students said they looked forward to the quality time with me. They saw that I could not work with everyone as closely as I should and that the shy students, as these two are, were getting the short end of the stick. I thought about my decisions a lot, but never too intensely. I've learned that sitting with an idea in your gut is the best way to determine if it's a good one. Sitting with an idea also gives space for new, better ideas to form.

I have come to realize that many of my reactions to my students' behaviors come from a place of my own previous trauma. It wasn't present in my conscious mind at that moment, but I had often reflected that these three young people reminded me of my brother. When I was 8, my family adopted my brother who was 15 at the time. He came from a life of constant trauma and instability. His arrival into my family developed in me a deep sense of compassion and nurturing at an early age. Through years of counseling, I have learned that it takes hard work to reverse the major damage some young people endure, and that even though my brother had to learn to be responsible for his actions, he often was not in control of them.

The most important tool I learned in counseling was grounded thinking and processing. I have learned how to sit with an idea and consult others before making decisions. I noticed that I was taking each situation too emotionally and personally. My successes throughout my tenure on the job were all rooted in my ability to do my job well regardless of the situation, including the student. I had the power, as the adult staff, to be the constant ingredient in every formula, yet I realized that I had become too triggered to think clearly enough to take rational action.

Carl, Dennis, and Julie have had complicated lives to say the least, but I have to always remind myself that they are still youth. Even though they have been forced to be independent in some ways, they are not in complete control of their lives yet. They need a compassionate, stable adult who will help them learn to take a firm grip on the reins. I was able, after some self-coaxing, to be that rational adult they needed to take control. I was able to continue as a positive figure in their lives.

I am proud that I was able to maintain my GED classroom's culture of learning and respect by giving each student an equal opportunity to study and grow as a young adult in a supportive environment. I know that I am ready to alter my program in any way, if necessary. Now students have more opportunity to engage with me and to focus. Some are not yet ready for this space; the door will be open for them when they are. Ultimately, I am proud that no one was punished for not being able to conform to a set of rigid classroom standards and that these students are back on the path to acquiring their diploma.

Unpacking the dilemma

These stories demonstrate just how challenging it is for youth workers to achieve the right balance between maintaining high standards for all youth and providing individualized support to achieve those standards. In the end, both youth workers decided to keep struggling youth in their programs in spite of them not adhering to program standards.

Both Melinda's and Loren's dilemmas exemplify how external factors affect young people's ability to participate fully in youth development programs. Vanessa struggles in school. Carl, Julie, and Dennis each have experienced difficult life events. Melinda and Loren have strong enough relationships with these youth that they are aware of their struggles. Both Melinda and Loren also have extremely high standards and approach their work with a great deal of intentionality. It is this combination of knowing the youth and knowing what they want them to get out of their programs that makes these situations so challenging. We now use the Ecological Dilemma Resolution model to analyze Melinda's and Loren's cases.

Knowledge

Both Melinda and Loren are relatively experienced youth workers. Melinda's career integrating youth development and the arts started when she was in high school and had the chance to work in a youth program that she had attended when she was a child. She has not stopped since. She developed her dancing and choreography skills in college. The demanding schedule she maintained while participating in three different dance teams and at the same time maintaining a strong performance in her classes taught her that balance between academics and the arts is possible. She experienced how participating in something she loves could feed her and keep her motivated when her studies got hard.

Unlike Melinda, Loren is not working in the community where she grew up. Rather, she came to the city to go to college. For Melinda, integrating arts and youth development was a natural path. Loren, on the other hand, always held an ambivalent stance toward formal education. While she understood that the young people in her GED program needed a diploma to get ahead in their lives, she always struggled with whether that was right or fair. Through counseling, Loren has learned strategies to help keep her grounded and maintain a healthy life/work balance. These strategies help her to consider multiple dimensions of complex problems before trying to solve them. She has learned that she needs to sit with ideas and consult with others before making decisions.

Dilemma Resolution Cycle

Problem identification

Melinda's immediate problem is whether to allow Vanessa to dance on the team, given that she is failing in school. Loren is facing a recurring problem with the behavior of a group of students in her GED class. Neither youth worker wants to add more burdens to the youth; yet they worry that they won't be doing these struggling youth, nor the other young people in their programs, any favors by bending the rules for them. Both Melinda and Loren realize that the reason these problems are difficult to resolve is that they are more deep and complicated than just needing to enforce rules.

Melinda often feels like she is the only one in the youth's lives who is conveying to them that they have to work hard, that there is a professional way that people expect things. She says it is hard to work against youth's upbringing and that sometimes she even feels like giving up. But the realization that she may be the only one telling them these things keeps her going and makes her question how she implements the standards for her program. Loren's ability to hone in on the problem was initially clouded by her strong negative emotional reaction to the possibility that Carl, Julie, and Dennis were coming back into her group. She realized that she had to understand why she was feeling triggered before she was able to attend effectively and compassionately to the needs of the youth.

Plan formulation

Melinda decided to let Vanessa continue to dance on the team because dancing was a source of positivity and pride in her life. Melinda concluded that Vanessa's improvements and connectedness outweighed the rule of getting passing grades to stay on the team. Melinda feared that excluding Vanessa would isolate her and cause her to withdraw again. Loren also felt that the youth who are most in need of her program struggle with the structure and expectations. Instead of making individual exceptions to the rules, however, she turns the problem on its head and restructures her whole program to better meet all of her students' needs.

Plan implementation

Once they decided what to do, both Melinda and Loren implemented their plans by sticking to what they devised with careful thought, intention, and belief that their plans would bring about the best outcome for the youth at hand.

Evaluation/reflection

Upon reflection, Melinda still feels that holding all youth to the same higher standard will help them more in the long run. Melinda does not want to punish youth—especially those who are already down. But she truly believes that her youth simply have to do better in order to make it in the world and that being too soft on the youth does them a disservice. Melinda voices doubts that her chosen course was the right thing to do and makes a vow for next year: "I have too much heart so they think they can get over on stuff. So next year I will be stricter on the grades from the beginning." Although she does wonder if she should account for individual circumstances, she feels that students will benefit more if she has more follow-through. Through reflection, Melinda turns evaluation into action in order to make revisions and continue learning. Melinda comes to the realization that while she may not have control over the youth's performance in school or family support, she does have control over her program. She believes she can structure it in a way that ensures youth can meet her expectations, even those coming from the most challenging situations.

Loren, on the other hand, realizes that she was taking the return of Carl, Julie, and Dennis too emotionally and too personally. When she started feeling triggered by the youth and unable to think rationally about what to do, she knew she had to sit with what was happening before making a decision. She remembered that as the adult staff, she had the power. She did not want to use her power *over* the youth to punish them for not adhering to her expectations. Rather she was able to put the youth's needs at the center of her thinking to reimagine her program in a way that would allow her to teach all students and increase the likelihood all students could learn.

REFLECTING ON PRACTICE:

What do Melinda and Loren do well in these stories? What strengths do they bring to youth work?

Where do they get stuck in their stories? What considerations are they balancing? In what ways are they similar and different?

Would you consider the decision of either youth worker to be the wrong one? Why or why not? Did either youth worker miss anything that they should have considered when making their decision?

In what ways can you relate to Melinda's and Loren's experiences? Have you ever been faced with the decision to enforce, bend, or break rules and standards for a young person you work with? What helped you make your decision? What were the implications of your decision?

Melinda acknowledges that it's sometimes the toughest kids who need someone to expect more of them and hold them to high standards. Yet when these young people don't meet the expectations set for them, what should the consequence be? How can youth workers keep these "tough" youth engaged and not isolate them further?

Summary

Melinda and Loren's dilemmas highlight how ecologically intelligent youth workers navigate the problem appraisal, evaluation, and reflection cycle. Through this reflective process, both youth workers question whether their programs are structured to best serve the youth who need it most. Eventually, they both decide to change the programs in some way to ensure the struggling youth can continue to participate. Melinda reflects a great deal on her program's standards and why she holds them, eventually deciding to relax the grade requirement so Vanessa can continue to dance with the team. However, the plan she formulates for next year is one where she will not let this happen again and will be stricter on her rules from the beginning.

Loren outlines in detail how she systematically restructured her class to ensure students' needs were met. The three youth who challenge Loren have difficult lives that affect their ability to participate in programs that are meant to help them.

Loren also recognizes that these young people have had to learn lessons the hard way all their lives and that what they really need is for someone to give them a chance. She sees the value in meeting youth in a place where they can all succeed with support and guidance from a responsible adult.

Digging deeper: applying the dilemma to your work

Activity 1: enforcing, bending, or breaking the rules

Imagine a youth work situation in which you were faced with a decision to enforce, bend, or break the rules for a youth.

- Describe the situation.
- How did you feel?
- What were you thinking?
- Why did that rule exist?
- What were the stakes if you decided to break the rule:
  - for the youth?
  - for your job/position?
- What were the stakes if you decided to enforce the rule:
  - for the youth?
  - for your job/position?
- What did you decide to do?
- Why did you decide to do that?
- What was the result?
- What would you do if you were in that situation again?

Activity 2: establishing group expectations and norms

When a group is forming, it is important to create a clear set of expectations that the group understands and respects. These expectations set norms for the group, help create a collective culture, and provide a grounding for how the group will function and progress. It is almost as if you are creating a "social contract" for the group to follow. Think about how you want these expectations to be constructed and utilized.

- Should the youth worker create and implement them?
- Should the youth have a hand in developing them?
- Which expectations might need to be written and which can be verbal?
- What can the youth expect from you as a leader?

Additionally, it is also good to remember to refer back to the expectations that were delivered at the beginning of your group's formation. If possible, have the youth group sign the agreements together or individually to reinforce accountability.

Expectations and how they are presented will obviously differ depending on the population you work with, the culture of your organization, your leadership style, and more. However, it is important to be mindful and intentional about both how and why expectations are created and further maintained.

Activity 3: reflecting on the role of adults in your childhood

Often the way we work with and interact with youth is a result of how we were treated by adults when we were growing up. Think of an adult in your life growing up that impacted your life positively and shaped your development.

- What was your relationship like with this person?
- Why did this person play an important role in your life?
- How do you know they cared about you?
- What expectations did they have of you?
- How did they communicate these expectations to you?
- In what ways do you think your relationship with this person affects your work with youth and/or your desire to work with youth?
- How can you remember how this adult made you feel when you are engaging with the youth in your programs?

5

BALANCING CONFLICTING VALUES FROM HOME, A YOUTH ORGANIZATION, AND THE COMMUNITY

Keeping youth well-being at the center of youth work

> *"I'm just a mirror. I'm here to help you sort things out, to reveal what you already know to be the best option for you and your future."*—Olivia

---

Chapter learning objectives

- Building deep and trusting relationships with youth
- Keeping youth's needs and well-being at the center of a youth worker's practice
- Drawing on resources and networks outside of one's organization

---

Youth workers often operate at the boundary between home, community, and their organization. Working in the context of deep and trusting relationships, youth workers have a unique glimpse into young people's lives. Due to their vantage point, youth workers often confront issues that "go beyond" the scope of their organization's mission, that can be in conflict with the youth's family's values, and that may challenge the youth worker's own beliefs. In these situations, youth workers are faced with moral dilemmas in trying to decide what to do with and for a youth.

This chapter explores such a dilemma involving Olivia, an experienced youth worker, and Darren, a program participant who wants to come out to his family as gay. Olivia works for College Prep, a four-year after-school leadership and college-access program. College Prep serves talented, first-generation, low-income students who are at risk of not attending college. Olivia acts as mentor to youth not only in an academic sense but also by helping to guide them through personal and family issues that may act as barriers to being able to go to college. Her background is similar to the youth she serves in that she is from an immigrant family. She was a teen mother and lived firsthand the struggles associated with completing high school and college. She was raised as an Evangelical Christian and this dilemma proved to challenge her own beliefs about homosexuality. In determining how to guide Darren, Olivia has to balance her own values, the mission of her organization, and the possible risks to the youth's relationship with his family.

Olivia interweaves her youth work philosophy and reflections into her telling of the dilemma story. Her rich narrative reveals a talented youth worker's thought processes and steadfast ability to keep a young person's well-being at the center of her work in spite of complex, competing forces surrounding the situation.

Olivia's story

Always at the first advising session and again when they leave I say: "I'm not your mom; don't be dependent on me. I am you; that's all I am. I am you. I am just a mirror. I asked you these questions and you answered them and you knew what you wanted the whole time."

I use the image of a mirror in explaining my job to the youth—that I'm like a reflection. I find that most of the time people already know the answer to their questions. They just need help feeling confident about it or helping it come out as a coherent thought. It's all scattered and they don't know how to read what's in their head, and I'm just helping—I'm just pulling it out for them and placing it in front of them. I let them know, "I will help you—I will help pull those things out, but those are *your* answers."

I try to engage youth with the idea of who they can become to get at the potential within them. We talk a lot and most of it, completely unintentionally, is very therapeutic based. My biggest role here is therapist even though we hardly even talk about it, but if you really break it down that's what it is. I have a couch, there are lots of tissues that have already been used up, and I sit in this chair and we sit in that one-hour session. During that time, I don't talk to them about their grades and resume, but more of: "How's your mom doing? How's this going? How's that problem you had last time?" You know the old saying you can't ask a hungry kid to study. The last thing they're thinking about is studying; the first thing they're thinking about is that immediate need to eat. That's how I think about emotional distress. If you're in emotional distress, how can I ask you to do anything else? Especially, worry about English class? So a lot of the things that we talk about are dealing with avoiding a midlife crisis. Youth don't understand the work that we're doing here is for when they're 40. I don't want them to find themselves in a place where they feel disappointment down the road.

I want to help young people make the best decisions, but I also want to raise expectations that they may not be used to, to expose them to new options. You hear a lot about people who have gone to college, have parents and grandparents that have gone to college, so that there's no question of *if* you are going to go to college. It's: "Where are you thinking about going? What are you thinking about studying?" In comparison, I think that so many people ask the young people I tend to work with: "Are you going to go to college?" I don't think that question ever comes to the table *here*. It's said right from the beginning that there is no failure; there are no other options here. You are with us or you're not and when you're here, you are *here*. I think that we don't give them the option not to go to college. I never use language that might ever give them the thought that there are other options. I use myself as an example of the idea there are so many places you can fail in life, and I talk to them about it and I expose them to other adults that they can relate to that are in that successful place.

Working with youth means working with families. Some families want to interact more with you and some, less; but having family interaction means aligning on goals. We've had pushback from families around life decisions that we're helping students make—like going away to college and not staying home. We see the need to allow young people to make those decisions for themselves, but sometimes I'm like, "this kid needs to get out of their house or else they're going to crumble." Should I be the one making the decision for them? What direction am I driving them in, intentionally, unintentionally?

Some of the kids we work with come from families whose attitudes we are fighting against—which I don't even know if we should be. I don't make decisions for them, but I'll ask a lot of questions. I had a student that I thought was limiting himself by trying to please his family and stay home instead of moving away for college. We worked through a lot of questions together. We processed the situation and got to the point where he could talk about what the best option for him would be. Again, *I'm* just a mirror and in that situation, I didn't make that decision for him; I just helped him to see his own answer. I want students to be able to answer the hard questions on their own because I'm not always going to be there; I don't want them to be dependent on me.

Dealing with family expectations about college and careers is one challenge, but we also see other conflicting beliefs and values outside of academic interests. For example, I had a student—Darren—approach me with a conflict. He wasn't even on my caseload but we had a lot in common. He could really identify with me and was comfortable with me. I was always hard on him; I wouldn't take excuses and instead just expected a lot of him, which actually built our relationship more. He had a lot of social struggles and felt like he had to be tough so he wouldn't get bullied. He was out as gay in our program and he was out at school, but he wasn't out at home. At school he was teased a lot. At our program, it was safer for him but there were still undertones from the males in the group. A lot of our conversations started out around how to avoid physical fights and dealing with kids who were bullying him.

Darren had not told me that he wasn't out to his family. I figured this out more from our discussions about feedback his family would give him about being too feminine—like sometimes he would paint his nails and they would say, "Why are you doing that?" or "Don't do that; you're going to give off the wrong impression." To me, it was so obvious; like, how could they not know? So there was some clear denial going on there. One day, he tells me he wants to come out to his parents.

I had never worked with GLBTQ students in any capacity and I was really invested in who he was and his journey because I had been working with him for three years at this point. Plus, I had seen Darren struggling and I was worried about him.

When I asked what he thought was going to happen, he said he already knew his family wouldn't accept it. I felt like I was in a little over my head so I reached out to my supervisor, who basically said we should tread with caution—that it wasn't our responsibility to coach him in this area. I also had a personal dilemma because I had spoken to my mom about it a few times and she would caution me also because it's not really accepted in our religion. My parents are really religious and I had grown up in that, but had formulated my own ideas. I was feeling really alone in this. My agency wasn't supporting me and the advice I was getting from the people I cared about wasn't really supportive either.

I went back to Darren and had a long discussion. I decided to go with my gut feeling and just tell him that he should do it. I figured that since he had brought it up to me and said he wanted to do it then I didn't think I was giving so much of my opinion, but more my support. I wasn't saying, don't do it or do it, but rather, if you feel like you should do it, I think you should do it. If it's weighing so heavily on you then that can't be healthy.

We talked about it maybe five more times over the course of about seven months until he finally came out to his parents. This was a very long process because he was so terrified, but within that process a lot of the things that came up let us share some of the weight that he had and now I had with his issue. We both picked up allies for support through this situation so we could both cope with it well and be a good support system to each other without overwhelming each other. It's not intentional, but sometimes when someone brings a problem to you, you end up dumping that problem back on them and you become part of the problem by feeling overwhelmed by what they just said to you. I was really scared that I would do that to him, so I needed to seek out outside support to deal with that.

Am I doing the wrong thing? Is this any of my business? What kind of authority do I have in giving any advice on this? I spoke to some of my friends who were out and talked to them about some of their experiences. What age did they come out? What was the worst thing that happened? What were their worst fears? I would bring these stories back to Darren, and it made me feel a lot better because over and over again I was getting that this was the right thing to do. Of course, I think everything youth workers do should be individualized and they should take the time to ask questions to get at young peoples' true motivations and wants. Sometimes it doesn't work and I feel scared or nervous, like when I think that things are dangerous for the student or I really don't know how to make a decision. Those are the times that I usually bring other people into the loop. I'm very comfortable receiving help and if we have two or three of us on board, we can come up with a reasonable solution that I didn't think of on my own.

The agency eventually found out I was doing all this work with Darren about his sexuality and his relationship with his family. They were pretty passive and very much took the stand of just refer him somewhere else; there are these groups that deal with that; let them work with him on this. But he knew about those groups and was even somewhat involved, and still he wasn't asking them these questions—he was asking me.

In the end, it was harsh when he told his parents and I was worried that he might be mad at me for encouraging him. He wasn't mad. He said it was pretty much the reaction he was expecting. Our conversations evolved into talking about seeking support and new challenges that arose as he graduated from the program and moved away.

It's been a journey for me as this all happened seven years ago. I'm still on that journey as the same issue comes up in other programs with other youth. I try to keep the youth at the center of the issue. They're involved in so many systems and getting so many messages, but ultimately they have to be able to make decisions for themselves. I keep reminding them and myself that I'm just a mirror. I'm here to help them sort things out, to reveal what they already know to be the best option for them and their future.

Unpacking the dilemma

Olivia is an insightful, empathetic youth worker who is deeply reflective and knows how to maintain her health so that she can be healthy for the youth. She navigates a risky path in her work with Darren. She recognizes the limitations in her personal knowledge, the lack of organizational support she has, and the possibility for danger and harm that could await Darren if coming out to his family goes poorly. She overcomes those limitations through two sets of actions. On the one hand, she goes deep with Darren. Through purposeful dialogue, she explores what Darren wants and probes to be sure he understands the complexity of the situation and the many possible outcomes of his coming out to his family. On the other hand, she fortifies herself. She reaches out to her network beyond her organization to learn as much as she can about how to support Darren through his process of coming out to his family. Her use of the mirror metaphor is emblematic of how she keeps the young person's well-being at the center of her work—as opposed to her own beliefs and values and the mission of her agency. We now use the Ecological Dilemma Resolution model to analyze Olivia's case.

Knowledge

Olivia has a well-developed praxis derived from her personal and practice knowledge. There are three basic tenets underlying her work. First, she believes strongly that youth's need for emotional health and support must come before they are able to focus on academic concerns. Olivia asks youth about their families, lives, and other concerns before she ever gets to the topic of their schoolwork or college futures. Second, she believes that young people have most of the answers they seek already inside themselves. Her role as youth worker is to help them pull those answers out of themselves. Third, she knows she must draw on the knowledge and experiences of others when she faces dilemmas that go beyond her own comfort level or area of expertise.

Dilemma Resolution Cycle

Problem identification

Olivia knows she must navigate a set of clashing values in determining what is best for Darren. Darren's family has problems with homosexuality. College Prep's core work is about helping first-generation students get into college; supervisors do not think Olivia should be working with Darren on how to come out to his family. Olivia even struggles to understand what her own beliefs are in this situation. Olivia navigates these conflicting dynamics by involving Darren in the whole process. She asks him hard questions and engages him in serious dialogue over the course of several months in order to understand what the central problem is.

Plan formulation

Just as Olivia is deliberate in working with Darren to identify the problem, she uses a similar process to formulate a course of action to support his decision to come out to his parents. Olivia communicates that youth cannot think about school when they are hungry, damaged, and in need of stability. While not disregarding the academic focus of her organization, Olivia knows that unless youth feel safe they won't be able to do the work they need to ensure a healthy future. She rejects the warnings of her employers to let another agency help Darren. Darren came to *her* with this need. Even though she feels over her head with this issue, she decides that she won't turn her back on him. She does not want to burden Darren with her own feeling of being overwhelmed by the situation. Instead, she fortifies herself by drawing on all the resources she can muster. She reaches out to friends who have come out as gay so that she can learn everything she can on what could happen when Darren comes out. She shares what she learns with Darren so he is more prepared.

Plan implementation

Darren and Olivia continue to dialogue about the issue over the course of seven months. Darren comes out to his family. It is horrible, but Darren survives with Olivia's continued support. They continue to work together on other issues in his life.

Evaluation/reflection

Olivia acknowledges that the dilemma with Darren was challenging and that she has faced similar dilemmas in the seven years since that happened. Olivia reflects on the importance of keeping youth at the center of the work at all times. Her stance has gotten her in trouble with the organizations she has worked for, but she does not waver from this stance.

REFLECTING ON PRACTICE:

What does Olivia do well in this story? What strengths does she bring to youth work?

Where does Olivia get stuck in this story? What keeps her from moving through the Dilemma Resolution Cycle?

Do you think Olivia made the best choices? How would you have approached the situation of Darren coming out to his family? How might this have turned out differently if she had pushed harder or quickened the pace of Darren's coming out?

What do think College Prep's concerns were about her handling LGBTQ identity issues herself? In what ways are these fears justified?

Can you relate to Olivia's experience? Have you ever been in a situation in which you had to juggle your beliefs and your organization's mission with what was ultimately best for the young person? How did you reconcile these tensions?

When is it best to refer a young person elsewhere? When is it harmful to the young person? What are the risks of referrals? What are the benefits?

Summary

Because of the dialogic nature of Olivia's approach with youth *before* dilemmas arise, she can focus on the needs and challenges facing young people before they become insurmountable problems. Olivia's attention to competing forces in a young person's life helps her to understand who they are and what going to college means to them. She cannot imagine helping them achieve that goal if other parts of their lives are unsettled or unsafe.

Family, school, friends, and relationships all create a dense system of ecological spaces that influence young people. Olivia's questions explore these realms and the role they play in a young person's life, making connections and helping them to navigate the obstacles they present. In exploring these systems, Olivia helps youth to overcome problems, heal disconnects, and gain access to resources formerly off limits or unknown. She engages with them about the challenges they face in their lives and introduces them to successful role models. Most important is that Olivia is breaking down barriers and creating new paths within the maze of life that youth may never have considered or had thought were beyond their abilities.

Yet she is not dictating the proper paths they should take. In the end, she works to create an empowered youth who can make these decisions for themselves with the maximum possible options and support of multiple systems. She teaches young people to do this for themselves; she equips them with the tools they need to untangle their needs, emotions, and issues and to tap into the knowledge they had all along to find their own answers. Sometimes her stance puts her in direct opposition to her organization's practices. Right or wrong, Olivia holds onto the idea that she is a mirror for the youth and that the core of her job is to help them reconcile the conflicting images they see in that mirror until the youth are whole and healthy. Olivia's approach to the dilemma reflects a deep understanding of youth work that combines ecological navigation of systems that conflict with youth empowerment, breaking down the barriers within these systems to discover paths for a self-determined future.

Digging deeper: applying the dilemma to your work

Activity 1: readying yourself to work with youth's challenges

Olivia stated, "Sometimes when someone brings a problem to you, you end up dumping that problem back on them and you become part of the problem by feeling overwhelmed by what they just said to you." When working with youth, there may be many difficult and upsetting situations that they bring to you and ask you to help them with. Some may be traumatic. Some may strike a personal chord within you. Some may feel like too much for you to handle. This is normal, and therefore it is necessary to have outlets for self-care and a network of resources so that the youth worker doesn't internalize the young person's situation and become less able to be a source of support.

Think of a situation when a youth has come to you for help and you felt overwhelmed by what they presented to you.

- Why did it feel overwhelming?
- What did the person need from you?
- Did you feel equipped to handle the situation?
- How did you handle the situation?
- What were you able to provide?
- Did you refer the person elsewhere?
- Did you have a support system to help you?
- What was the outcome?

Think of what self-care means to you.

- Why is self-care important when working with youth?
- What de-stresses you?
- What types of self-care measures do you take?
- In what ways can you seek help from others as a form of self-care?

Consider to what extent your organization was supportive when a young person needed additional help.

- Think about and list the requirements of your organization.
- List all the tools you can or may already use for keeping youth at the center of your work.
- Now, consider how these two realms of your work may come in conflict with one another and keep you from being able to fulfill your requirement and/or keep youth at the center.
- Brainstorm ways to balance organizational requirements so that you can maintain a young person's needs and well-being at the center of your work.

Activity 2: building your network

Make a list of providers, programs, and agencies that you have worked with and/ or most commonly refer youth to.

- What is your relationship like with these other providers?
- How do you maintain your relationship so you can connect in the future?
- What resources might not be on your list that could be useful? Are they not on your list because they don't exist? Or are they not there because you haven't established a connection with the provider yet?
- How can you reach out to develop relationships with additional community partners?

6

YOUTH WORKER AND ORGANIZATIONAL RESPONSES TO RISKY BEHAVIOR AND DANGEROUS SITUATIONS

Chapter learning objectives

- Being able to think on your feet while staying calm and focused on the dangerous situation at hand
- Assessing youth moods and behaviors and taking appropriate action
- Knowing and using your organization's policies

Community-based youth organizations should be spaces where youth are safe from physical and emotional violence and should be places where young people learn strategies to resist risky and illicit behavior. Yet reality can interfere with this ideal. Adolescence is a time of experimentation. As youth workers, we try to minimize the harm of their inevitable experimentation with drugs, sexual activity, and challenging rules—but we can't prevent all risky behavior. We also need to realize that as youth workers, we have limited ability to *change* youth and where they come from. Young people develop their identity and decision-making processes in families, peer groups, neighborhoods, and schools. Youth organizations can play a role in helping young people make good choices, but youth workers need to understand that they are competing with other complex forces.

In this chapter, we hear two youth worker stories. William and Rebecca are forced to balance the interests of young people involved in risky behavior with the safety and well-being of other young people in their programs. Both stories present the challenge of thinking on your feet in the face of youth's risky behavior.

Introducing William and Rebecca

William is a white youth worker who came to the city where he now works five years ago. His journey started in New Hampshire but he spent most of his childhood in South Carolina, where his analysis of race and power began. He realized he wanted to be an educator when he was in middle school. He credits early experiences in school with fueling his desire to facilitate young people's learning:

> I had teachers who encouraged a lot of learning. People like to criticize the South for not being as far along as the North in terms of racial equality. I shoot back: "How many teachers of color did you have growing up? 'Cause I had a lot and they were the strongest, most memorable teachers I had."

He gave a great deal of thought to the type of educator he wanted to be and realized non-formal, community-based work matched his values and work style. He works at a youth leadership development program that focuses on college readiness for first-generation college-goers.

Rebecca is part of a small nonprofit organization that focuses on urban environmental and social justice. This organization runs a youth leadership program that has shared power and consensus-based decision-making as core principles. Youth are on the board and are co-directors with equitable responsibility, power, and compensation to adults in the organization. Youth teach youth wherever possible, using a community organizing model that upholds the belief of not doing for anyone what they can do for themselves. The adults who formed this group believe that youth involvement is a way of "waking the youth up to their agency, to their individual and collective power." But Rebecca notes that: "Often youth lean on adult staff for guidance and input. We want them to have the full opportunity to exercise their power and good judgment, but they often look to us for authority." Rebecca is in her late twenties. She came to the community where she now works to go to college. She is very familiar and comfortable with consensus-based organizations. Her uncle is a professional mediator who, in his work in criminal justice, utilizes restorative justice processes that include all parties at the table. About her uncle's work, Rebecca says, "I've watched him have his heart broke a number of times, but he keeps at it."

Her prior work with organizing former prisoners taught her a lot about how poor decisions as a young person can negatively affect a person's life. But because she has also seen people change their decision-making patterns—make better choices and live healthier lives—she deeply believes in harm reduction instead of incarceration. She describes herself as "straight edge" [strictly substance free] due to her strict upbringing and seeing what addiction has done in the lives of many close friends. Because she is multiracial, she feels people often assume she is more of an insider than she actually is.

William's dilemma

We were about to start our regular group meeting; two youth, Jade and Carolina, roll into the meeting about five minutes late. It was immediately apparent that they were preoccupied. I got the meeting started, but they were very disruptive. The two eventually got up and went to the bathroom. Another girl took that opportunity to whisper to me that Carolina was going to get into a fight that afternoon at Crestview Park. I was like, "okay, a fight is being planned and a place has been chosen, but she's in the meeting so she isn't fighting right now."

I felt like I had to keep the meeting going to keep the girls' attention from the fight. But as the meeting went on, Carolina became increasingly distracted. Her cell phone kept going off and at one point I grabbed it and said, "I think that's distracting you." Carolina said, "okay, okay, okay." That lasted for a few minutes, at which point she got up from the meeting to go to the bathroom again. On her way out, I guess she grabbed her phone, although I hadn't noticed that. When she came back to the meeting, she was acting even more erratic. She just burst into the meeting and said, "I gotta go; my mom just called and I gotta go!" I said: "You are interrupting the meeting; why don't you just stay? Tell your mom you need five more minutes 'cause the meeting's almost over." And Carolina said, "I don't wanna wait; I just gotta go!" I told her to sit down. Finally she said "okay" and sat down.

We had a final question to discuss in small groups. During that exercise, Carolina must have gotten up and left. I had not realized it because I was working with another group. When I noticed she was gone, I sent another student to see if she was still around but students were telling me that she and Jade had left the building. I thought to myself, "okay, obviously she didn't go with her mother, and Jade is gone too." I ended the meeting and ran down to the park. On my way down, I found Carolina and Jade walking up the street. Carolina's face was bloody. I asked her if she was okay; she said, "yeah, yeah I'm fine." And at that point she told me what was going on.

On the way to the meeting that day, Carolina and Jade had run into a girl they call Frankie. Frankie had been harassing Carolina at school and repeatedly made threatening phone calls to her telling her, "you need to get away from my ex-boyfriend; he's cheating on you anyway." This run-in before the meeting got her really upset. Carolina said she was at a breaking point, where she was like: "Fine, I'll fight you—that's it. If it'll get you off my back, I'll fight you." So they set up the fight at Crestview Park.

But when Carolina and Jade got there, there were two carloads of people. Apparently Frankie's mom and aunt drove her to the fight and brought others to watch. As they were telling me the story, I was thinking to myself, "wow, so the mom and the aunt were approving of this." According to Carolina and Jade, these women also kept it a one-on-one fight, but not to Carolina's benefit.

Carolina has a bum shoulder that frequently goes out of place, so when she went to throw a punch she threw her shoulder out. The pain drove her to the ground. Frankie then took her and slammed her face down. Jade, who is not the fiery type that gets into fights, came over and pushed Frankie off Carolina. But Frankie's mom grabbed Jade's hair and was like, "this is a one-on-one fight"; but at that point, Frankie's sister was beating up Carolina.

As I was gathering all this information, Carolina's and Jade's parents came. Carolina's mom was very upset. She didn't know if she should call the school or the police or just leave it alone. I let her know that if a student gets in a fight after school—especially if it started in school—then the students would get suspended. We talked about why no one in school had done anything about this, especially because the problem had been brewing for a while. The girls told us that the school had had a mediator but that she had recently been laid off due to budget cuts.

When I talked to Carolina later that night, she said that she and her parents decided that they were not going to do anything about the incident; they were just going to "bury it." Carolina would stay out of school for a few days and let everything calm down. I was dubious. I reminded her that there had been two carloads of people and that her face was really banged up, with stitches over her eye. Carolina then admitted that the whole thing had been videotaped and the sisters threatened that they would be putting it on YouTube. I did not see how this would stay quiet, and I did not think it was the right thing to do anyway. But Carolina was adamant against pressing charges or bringing it up to anyone with authority at school. She said she would lie about how she got injured—say that she "fell off her uncle's motorcycle." I told her that if I heard that as a teacher, I would say there's no way that's what happened. I said that there's another way that we might be able to handle this. I said we could maybe get a community mediator. Carolina and her family agreed to this, but Frankie's family never responded to the request.

William's reflection

So, that's the dilemma I was in. You can see the kind of layers of choices that I made or didn't make. Looking back, I'm doubting some of what I did. I was informed enough to interrupt the situation more than I did. And I wonder if I ran to the park and it was still going on, what would I have done? I realized that I wasn't actually thinking about that. I didn't think about calling the police. I didn't tell anybody at my organization that I had left the building to break up a fight. I was just like, "I gotta go; I gotta go see what is happening." So I'm questioning— maybe I should have told somebody; maybe they could have been more effective. But these are the things I thought of after the fact.

Rebecca's dilemma

I notice the smell of pot as I pick them up. But I don't mention it, hoping it's coming from outside the car. At the meeting they are not themselves. At first they are all giggles. Normal things are hilarious. Before long, they're sleepy. Then one eats sunflower seeds till she says her mouth aches. At this point, I am 95 percent sure that they are stoned. I furiously cling to the remaining 5 percent of doubt because I don't want to believe that they are already disrespecting the workplace, having signed the collective agreements to be sober at work just two weeks ago. Plus there is no "hard evidence" and calling for a urine test is not an option. We don't want to get into the relationship of a suspicious boss.

I was furious and not sure what to do. I knew a timely response was critical. I had seen things progress quickly to a very bad place when blind eyes were turned to substance use in the workplace. I was also aware that a different youth worker might have pulled the girls right out of session and sent them home. But I knew myself. I needed time to watch the situation unfold to devise the best response.

I knew that one of the girls—Lia—was in an extremely vulnerable place. She had had some trouble with the law. Because of her rocky relationship with her mother, she had just been put in foster care. She had been through drug rehab. Through her brother, I knew that Lia has been involved in neighborhood gang activity. The other girl—Julissa—had only been with the group for two weeks and was too new in the group to have built a trusting relationship with me.

By the end of the day I was ready to address their subpar participation and to hint at the drug use by reminding them that *being ready for work* was part of the collective agreement they had signed on to. In the car ride back I told the girls we had to talk. But the girls were eager to leave, so we agreed to push the whole discussion to the next day.

I was okay with delaying the discussion. I figured we could use a Community Meeting, our organization's process, to address these types of situations. Although drug use is personal, I reasoned that the violation of the collective agreement was certainly the business of the group. Any youth or staff could call a Community Meeting to resolve a conflict or pass an urgent proposal. Youth and adults are trained (by youth and adults) to facilitate these meetings and are also trained in conflict resolution. All decisions are made by consensus in which all members, even those seen as responsible for a problematic situation, have an equal say and the power to halt the progress of any proposal. Usually one person presents their view of a situation, others involved directly respond, and then everyone is given the chance to speak until nobody has anything left to say and resolution has been reached. This process is informed by restorative justice.

I spent a lot of time that night discussing the details of the situation with my partner. I came to realize that the pot use in the workplace was *THE* core issue and had to be addressed. The more I talked about it, the more I was able to let go of that 5 percent doubt. I knew I had to be careful constructing my proposal for the Community Meeting. I felt all the youth needed a bold reminder that drug use is absolutely not an option at work, and at the same time, I wanted to respect the collective governance of the group. I put together the following proposal:

1   I'm calling a Community Meeting because I have to make a proposal I don't want to make.

2   Julissa and Lia—I know and you know that you appeared stoned at our session yesterday.

3   Just two weeks ago you signed off on our code of conduct, stating that you would maintain a 100 percent sober workplace and you would always be prepared for work.

4   Not maintaining these internal policies affects: a) the productivity of our group, b) the health of our members (you), c) the reputation of our group, d) the culture of our workspace.

5   Because you have violated the policies created by our group, I propose to fire you once we've paid you for your time with us, excluding yesterday when you were stoned.

6   I don't want to make this proposal because I know the energy, talent, and passion that you both can bring to the group—that's why we hired you both hands down. I've seen your A game. But unfortunately you made the decision to bring your Z game to work yesterday.

7   Whatever it is that causes you to behave as you did yesterday is something you will have to get to the root of to be successful in your lives. But you can't bring this group down with you.

While I felt ready, the next day did not go exactly as I had planned. Before work, Lia texted me to apologize for her lack of participation the day before; she said that she had had a really bad headache. I figured that she knew a serious proposal was brewing. The apology did cool some of my frustration, even though I didn't really believe the excuse. At least Lia was aware her behavior was off.

The Community Meeting I called didn't happen till late in the day. I was hoping to have it first thing but the people who needed to be in the room for it were not there at the same time. Then, when we finally had the Meeting, the youth facilitator of the workday chose to place it late on the agenda. When I was finally up, I started by pulling out the group-created contract that both the girls had signed two weeks before. I had them read it. Lia and Julissa were defensive and one of them stopped and said "ooooh" on the line about being sober at work. They both denied being high; their excuses were that they have been friends since fourth grade so they get goofy together and that one had been awake till 4 in the morning the previous night, and a third girl pointed out that she knew one was being screened periodically for drugs so she couldn't have been high.

Several members expressed that they understood why the issue was so important but that they wished they had been there to witness the situation for themselves. The one boy who had been in the car with them said he didn't notice anything. He had grown up with these girls and I thought he was probably covering out of fear or loyalty. He was also a new hire, unfamiliar to the group's process. I felt that he is very clearly the type to choose the path of least resistance and avoid confrontation.

Eventually everyone, including the girls, understood why I was proposing what I proposed; why I was bringing up what I was bringing up. Everyone reaffirmed that the group policies for and by the group HAD to be respected. But the girls would not admit to the drug use, so I backed down. I let my proposal to fire them slide, and I apologized for my accusation. The group seemed to be ready to move on with the understanding that drugs and not being prepared for work is taken VERY SERIOUSLY by me and the team.

Lia remained heated during the rest of the Meeting but said she was good by the end of it. She was pretty cheery at the end of the day. Both girls were singing when they did their timesheets. They stopped singing or dancing whenever I looked their way. I realized that Lia wouldn't be over this any time soon. I was sad that our relationship might be challenged. My coworker Jack tried to reassure me that I did the right thing. He said:

> Maybe she can't like you right now. She is incredibly defensive about this kind of thing because she is getting it from all sides of her life: family, foster home, school, etc. I guess one more place where she knows she has to be sober is a good thing, even if it frustrates her.

Rebecca's reflection

Although my proposal to fire the girls did not go through, I was actually happy with the outcome. I expected there would be lots of resistance to the proposal. But I also knew that to sweep it all under the rug and not bring it up would have had a terrible impact on our group. Hopefully keeping the girls on the team doesn't encourage them or others to use drugs. Since that Community Meeting, this issue has not come up again. I am happy to not have the feeling of "waiting for the next time" heavy in my gut, which I know would be there if it had not been brought up in the Meeting. And I'm even more happy that within a few weeks Lia and I were back in a good space.

Unpacking the dilemma

William navigates dangerous terrain. The youth he works with are embroiled in a situation that has escalated from verbal harassment to physical conflict and violence. He does not utilize his organization's protocols in handling this situation; in fact, we never learn if his organization has a protocol. Instead, he acts alone to try to resolve this dilemma. Using this approach, William learns about the complexity of the situation after the fight has already happened. He manages to talk to Carolina and her family but this further complicates what to do about the conflict with the girls. In considering the pros and cons of involving the police, the school, the community-based mediators, the other family, the youth organization, and the young people, William must weigh possible solutions and how they could lead to unanticipated negative outcomes for both Carolina and Frankie.

Unlike William, Rebecca works within the structures her organization has developed to handle breaches of protocol. Rebecca's organization has rules that are created and agreed to by youth, generally making ownership and adherence to these rules much more commonplace. Rebecca believes that Lia and Julissa violated these rules by coming to work high. Rebecca must balance enforcing rules, her own doubts about whether the youth are really high, and her knowledge of the life challenges Lia faces. She also has to consider how her own straight-edge beliefs mesh with her commitment to using restorative justice principles. Successful navigation of these tensions can lead to transformative youth work, yet a misstep at any point could potentially lead to alienating youth who most need to be in youth development programs.

Knowledge

William is a relatively experienced youth worker who works comfortably in a non-formal education framework. As a white man who grew up in the South, he has a unique perspective on race and education. He is keenly aware of the implications of involving law enforcement in issues related to youth of color.

Rebecca has both witnessed and practiced restorative justice processes. She firmly believes that young people should not suffer long-term consequences for typical youth mistakes. She also firmly believes that substance abuse in the workplace needs to be addressed quickly—both for the sake of the individuals involved in drug use and for the health and productiveness of the workplace.

Dilemma Resolution Cycle

William faces a series of dilemmas that unfold in part due to his actions and inactions at each decision point. Below, we focus on the first part of his dilemma. We ask you to analyze other decision points using the Dilemma Resolution Cycle below.

Problem identification

William is able to identify the problem facing him in his classroom: Carolina is getting ready to fight another girl later that day.

Rebecca recognizes the drug use issue right away, but second-guesses herself as she delves into the complexities of Lia's relationship to the justice system and her own fear of creating an authoritarian relationship with youth. She later solidifies her identification of the problem by talking with her partner and reflecting on past similar dilemmas.

Plan formulation

William tries to use the group meeting as a distraction for the girls. He believes that if he can just keep them in the meeting, they won't be fighting.

Rebecca considers how to respond that day to the youth misconduct. But Rebecca doesn't want to create a dynamic where she becomes the "suspicious boss" who demands drug testing and other policies that negatively control and impact youth. This is especially true in Rebecca's perspective on Lia who is already facing similar control by foster systems, legal systems, and rehab programs. Here

Rebecca stalls, but falls back on her knowledge of restorative justice from her work with ex-prisoners and her uncle. She manages to work through her feeling surrounding betrayal and her fear of making a mistake, and seeking support from her coworkers and partner creates a proposal that holds the youth accountable yet still gives youth autonomy over the final decisions within the cooperative. Rebecca struggles to build the energy to propose firing both Lia and Julissa for their direct breach of collective agreements. She realizes she is taking an extreme position, but her proposal clearly lays out her reasoning. While this case may have been better resolved with an individual warning on the day of the infraction, Rebecca's proposal sends a clear message.

Plan implementation

William holds steadfast to his plan to keep Carolina and Jade in the meeting and to minimize distractions for the rest of the group. He takes Carolina's phone. He refuses to allow them to leave to meet Carolina's mom. Yet his work facilitating the group did not allow him to put his full attention to Carolina and Jade, and as a result, they were able to leave the meeting and go to the park to fight.

Rebecca was able to keep calm enough throughout her interaction and meeting with the girls, although she was fuming inside. She felt disrespected, disappointed, and angry; yet she remained logical and focused on the best way to approach the youth and continued to act calmly even when they argued with her and became defensive. If she had been more reactive, the girls may have become even more upset than they were. The group blocks the proposal from going forward, and so the consequences essentially remain a warning to the group about workplace standards, mutual responsibility, and the serious nature of collective agreements.

Evaluation/reflection

In hindsight, William sees the things he let slip through the cracks in the heat of the moment. He questions what would have happened if he had let his organization know right away that trouble was brewing. Would there have been support or a guideline that could have helped him navigate this experience? He realizes he did not have a plan about what he was going to do when he got to the park. He wonders if he could have intervened with them directly and immediately at the meeting as a means of stopping the fight. After the fact, he thinks he probably should have sacrificed the effectiveness of the group meeting to keep the girls safe.

Ultimately, Rebecca is pleased with the outcome of her intervention with Lia and Julissa. Although she may have been better off talking with the girls on the day she suspected they were high, the collective nature of the group supported her in holding the girls to community agreements. Rebecca feared the proposal to fire the girls would damage her relationship with the youth. She was also concerned that not going through with the proposal could signal to the youth that drug use would be tolerated. Neither fear was realized, however, as Rebecca was able to re-establish her relationship with the girls and there hadn't been another incident of a youth using drugs on the job.

REFLECTING ON PRACTICE:

What do William and Rebecca do well in their stories? What strengths do they bring to youth work?

Where do they get stuck? What keeps them from moving through the Dilemma Resolution Cycle?

Neither William nor Rebecca directly confronted the youth in their stories when they felt something was amiss. Could these situations have unfolded differently if the youth workers had immediately sat the youth down individually and asked them what was going on? Was there any benefit to waiting in either story? Explain.

What are your organization's policies and protocols on fighting and drug use? How useful would they have been in these cases? What makes it easy or hard to enforce them?

In what ways can you relate to William's and Rebecca's experiences? Have you ever had to make a quick decision about handling youth risk behavior? What considerations did you weigh? What decision did you come to? What was the outcome of your decision? Would you do something differently next time you are in a similar situation?

Summary

An immediate dilemma that presents itself concerns where William's job ends and someone else's begins. Is William responsible for the conduct of his youth outside of his youth program? Is it his place to navigate the difficult dynamics and relationships with school, the legal system, community mediation, and a complicit family with which he has no past relationship? There are few easy answers to such questions, and perhaps this case study reaches into uncharted territory in which youth workers frequently find themselves. Youth workers are often major players in young people's lives beyond the confines of their job description or program, but go largely unsupported in this capacity.

Directly confronting Carolina about the situation, especially given a prior relationship, may have altered the situation into one in which both youth worker and youth could create a mutual solution—if only temporarily. However, the violence here is much more complex than a one-off fight. At what point does a youth worker pass the buck off to another player in the ecological web? This situation can often arise in even simple dilemmas. A youth worker may feel lost in the midst of action, only to find there is simply no one to pass the buck to. This can leave youth workers exposed and burnt out. In this case, William is working closely with Carolina and her mother to come up with solutions, but finds the wishes of Carolina and her family to be working at cross-purposes to achieving a long-term solution. Will the fights continue if no legal recourse is sought? Will social media footage of the fight escalate the harassment into new levels? When and how will the school become involved? Carolina's family seeks to keep these system players out of the solution, leaving William as the only non-familial professional to advocate for youth-centered solutions.

Rebecca quickly moved from identification of the problem to deciding to use an established organizational procedure for addressing conflict. Although she second-guessed her methods and whether she should move forward, her experiences of past drug-related dilemmas led her to act in a timely manner. By consulting her partner and coworker, she was able to process the dilemma and her own feelings about it into a formalized plan that she brought to the youth. Together they addressed the issue in light of collective agreements on appropriate behavior, which upset the youth yet served as a functional reminder about the seriousness of the workplace standards. Overall, Rebecca was able to move through the dilemma based on supportive organizational structures and staff as well as past experience and belief systems.

Digging deeper: applying the dilemma to your work

Activity 1: thinking on your feet (part two)

The ability to *think on your feet* actually requires a great deal of preparation. You need to know about the resources at your disposal and your organizational protocols, and have time to plan ahead. Take time to familiarize yourself with your organization's rules and standards of behavior, as well as the consequences of rule breaking. What should you do in case of fights? In case of theft? Drug use? What resources do you have beyond these protocols to refer youth to?

- Talk to other youth workers in your organization or area to see how they would have handled William's and Rebecca's dilemmas. How have they handled major dilemmas in the past?
- Make a resource list for yourself as you answer these questions.

By preparing ahead of time, you will have a better sense of how to engage quickly and effectively with these issues in the heat of the moment.

Activity 2: reflecting with others

It is important in youth work to remember to learn from other youth workers. Use the Dilemma Resolution Cycle to analyze what you would have done in the dilemma William faced. In particular, what would you have done once you realized the girls had left the building? After you have written down your own ideas, read the reactions of three other youth workers to William's dilemma, given below.

What are the possible consequences of these different approaches? How does their analysis mesh with your own? In what ways are they different? Would their methods work in your own organization? How does the input of other youth workers inform or improve your own dilemma cycles and analysis?

Youth Worker Response #1:

> If something like that happens at our organization, we just call the police. But you know calling the general tip line is a crapshoot 'cause if the kids aren't fighting when they come then you sent them on a false call. But we have a great relationship with the gang unit, so we call the gang unit and say two kids are gonna fight at this spot at this time. We give them a heads-up and they get there while things are happening. The kids see police and it kind of squashes stuff. You gotta squash it because with the anti-bullying laws … and then this stuff pops up on Facebook—if they weren't going to press charges before, now you're definitely going to have to press charges.

Youth Worker Response #2:

> I've been in a situation like that before where we had a relationship with kids and we could see the fight brewing. You see the girls talking; you see the cell phones out. I jump in and say: "You wanna tell me what's going on? I'll follow you home if I have to." For me, everything stops, and so I know this girl is not going to fight, at least right now. And normally it'll come out, and she'll say something like "well she wants me to meet her there." I tell her "you're not going to meet her there later." These kinds of techniques to avoid this kind of situation as a quick fix … but once that was done, that's kind of where we fell short. You can't be with them all the time. And also talking to her and giving her the skills to avoid the fight or whatever probably gets at the heart of what really is between her and this girl. I mean she could have been doing a number of things to bring this kind of heat on herself that would be addressed. You know—"What are you doing? What's going on that's making this fight?"

Youth Worker Response #3:

> One thing I've noticed is that when we talk about the dilemmas, we often start at the black and white. … We started at the place of "to suspend or not-suspend, to get rid of her or not get rid of her." And then it gets deeper and deeper. … We started with "to call the police or not" but then it got more complex. What I also found interesting is that things like these anti-bullying laws have enormous potential to harm young people. Yet all the supports that could help mediate this are eliminated. I just wonder where will the youth worker's job end? I would help the family find a culturally sensitive mediator but if that doesn't work, where do I go from there? Do we talk to the school administration? It may go on forever, with little to no support from the rest of the organization.

7

BALANCING YOUTH PRIVACY WITH THE YOUTH WORKER'S NEED FOR INFORMATION

The importance of organizational support in dilemma resolution

"If I had only known she hadn't taken her medication that morning, the whole day could have been different."—Katie

Chapter learning objectives
- Knowing how to navigate and negotiate organizational policies
- Understanding the need for a "plan B" when tried-and-true strategies are not working
- Utilizing appropriate lines of communication within an organization to resolve dilemmas

An organization's structure, mission, values, and policies can set the stage for how youth workers are able to serve young people. Organizations must provide sufficient training, support, and access to the resources they need, and a reasonable workload (Dennehy *et al.*, 2006). Organizations can support their youth workers through a range of practices including providing social and emotional support, and encouraging communication and debriefing when issues arise. Youth workers need to be able to seek additional help, if they need it, and not feel as though they are completely on their own. Building social and emotional support into the goals of the programs makes for better-quality programs (Khashu and Dougherty, 2007).

Organizational support can be resources youth workers have available to them, often in the form of funding, supplies, and other staff members or volunteers; but it can also be access to information on youth medical conditions, difficult life experiences, and necessary accommodations. Youth workers are best able to respond to dilemmas if they have all possible tools at their disposal. Organizations that value youth workers as professionals create an environment of communication and trust that can be achieved by creating channels of communication between different levels of staff, where front-line staff feel heard and have access to information. Programs must balance the various rights and needs of their youth with the goals of the organization. At times, multiple goals can be in conflict with each other—like maintaining confidentiality of client information and maintaining youth emotional and physical safety.

This chapter introduces a dilemma that Katie, a camp counselor, confronted in her one-to-one work with a camper, Amy, who had special needs. The organization in this chapter does offer training and a reasonable workload, but the support and access to resources (in this case information) is called into question.

The dilemma arose on the last day of an inclusive summer camp. After two weeks during which Katie was developing a caring relationship with Amy, on the last day of camp, the camper has repeated meltdowns, leading Katie to have to discipline her. When one of the episodes leads Katie to bring Amy to the Camp Director, she learns that Amy's parents forgot to provide the Camp Nurse with enough medication for the last day. This case raises issues about working with young people who have special needs and how an organization's policy about only sharing essential information with staff in order to preserve the privacy of youth can have unintended harmful consequences for the youth.

Introducing Katie

During the summer of 2013, I worked at Camp Mayfield, an inclusive summer camp. "Inclusive," for Camp Mayfield, means that it is designed for children with and without special needs, and there is a pretty even split between the two populations. The camp operated as an overnight and day camp, and I was working in the overnight part of the camp, meaning I was with the campers from early Sunday afternoon to late Friday afternoon. We did all the "normal" camp activities: horseback riding, swimming, archery, crafts. Everything was able to be modified to suit the needs of any participant, making a truly holistic experience for any camper who visited.

Camp Mayfield is committed to treating all students as similarly as possible. The camp is a non-restraint facility, so while the nature of some children's disabilities may make them prone to violent or dangerous behaviors, staff are never allowed to put their hands on them, even if they are trying to get them out of a potentially harmful situation. The camp takes confidentiality very seriously. Any information that isn't vital to share with other staff or those outside of camp will not be distributed. This includes campers' medical history, special needs, or anything else that may violate their privacy. This policy is followed very strictly by administrators and they enforce it with little flexibility.

I had never planned to work at an inclusive camp or with youth who had disabilities. I had been desperately searching for a summer job. Nothing was coming through. My father reminded me about Camp Mayfield, which was only about 45 minutes from my home. I applied, but I have to be honest—I was a bit scared to work with this population. I was afraid I would not be able to do a good enough job providing for them. But I told myself I could adapt and learn and that if I got the job, everything would be alright.

After getting the job, I committed myself to creating a loving, supportive environment that catered to the needs and abilities of all of my campers. I've always believed that everybody deserves the same treatment, regardless of the characteristics that so often dictate our experiences, like gender, race, and class. I wanted to create a space where disability would not define any of the youth, like it sadly so often does in places outside of camp. I quickly saw that camp was a safe haven for the kids. Not only did they feel like they belonged but they also felt happy. It was so easy to see it in their smiles and their laughter. So while I had never done any work with children with special needs, I immediately felt tied to the camp's mission and wanted to do my best to uphold it. Even though the work was hard, I felt like I was giving back to my community in a way that was so desperately needed.

My first week was particularly challenging. I had been paired with Matthew one-to-one for the whole week, based on the amount of attention he needed. One-to-one campers are included with the entire group but have one counselor working directly with them so that they are given as much support and attention as possible. He was difficult to work with. He didn't want to go to any activities. He regularly cursed at me. He became physically violent. It seemed he just didn't like camp. Try as I may, I felt like I wasn't making much headway with him. By the end of the week, I was ready to accept defeat. I brought him to his last horseback riding lesson, hoping for the best but bracing myself for the worst. As we talked on our way down to the stables, I decided to take a shot in the dark and ask him about his favorite part of camp. To my surprise, he answered willingly and enthusiastically: "Now I feel more confident and like I can do anything." In that moment, I felt like I had done my job. But more than that, as a human being I felt like I had a meaningful interaction with another person. I also learned an important lesson about youth work: none of this young person's anger was directly my fault or directed at me. I thought about his life outside of camp, living with special needs. I thought about how he processed information differently from most other children. I began to understand more deeply how this camp was supporting him. These insights helped me through five more weeks at Camp Mayfield.

Over that summer, thanks to experiences like the one I had with Matthew, I came to love this job. It was difficult and frustrating. But seeing a camper become brave enough to sing at talent show or confident enough to hold an archery bow on their own made the job rewarding over everything else. I had worked both in groups and in other one-to-one situations. My supervisors had seen me handle challenging situations and gave me some positive feedback on my approach. And so, when they sat me down and told me I would be working one-to-one with Amy during the last two weeks of the summer, I felt confident I could handle it. They assured me I'd love Amy and that they had a good feeling about our pairing.

When Amy arrived on Sunday, however, I immediately felt in over my head. My confidence quickly evaporated. One of my first experiences with her was her running away, outside and into a thunderstorm, when my back was turned. As I ran looking for her in the heavy rain, panicking that something bad would happen, it was instantly clear to me that working with Amy for two weeks would test my patience and dedication to this job.

Katie's dilemma

I spent most of the first week with Amy trying to figure out what set her off, what calmed her down, and what she responded to. For example, I quickly saw that Amy loved the pool and that she behaved most of the time she was swimming. But the minute I had to tell her it was time to leave the pool, she would have a meltdown. Sometimes they were just mild, but other times she put herself and others in danger, like when she would get mad at other campers for invading her personal space and lash out at them. We had developed a sort of unspoken system between the two of us and it was visibly working. As long as I could pull Amy away from potential meltdown situations quickly enough and do something else she enjoyed, she remained happy. We would spend a lot of time away from the group, doing whatever made her happy in the moment, and I grew to relish the one-on-one time. It made me understand how to respond to Amy and how to interact with her and realize what a bright, loving child she was. She was having fewer meltdowns, was being more cooperative, and seemed generally happy. I was expecting our last day together to go as smoothly as the previous ones had gone and was looking forward to making my last bit of time with her as meaningful as possible.

However, on this last day of camp, Amy had been having meltdown after meltdown. As I sat with the lifeguard and watched her swim, we talked about it. Maybe Amy just was sad to be leaving and didn't know how to express those feelings. Maybe she was in some sort of pain she didn't know how to describe. Because Amy could only express her emotions in very simplistic terms, it was left up to me to gauge the situation as best I could.

At the end of swim lessons, I asked Amy to get out of the pool, but she ignored me and kept swimming. When she finally got out of the pool, I took out her behavior chart. The behavior chart was a tool from her parents to reinforce positive behavior. For each activity Amy did well in, she earned TV time back at home. For each she did poorly in, she received an X on her chart as well as any related consequence. I told her that as a consequence of her actions, she would be losing five minutes of pool time later in the day. She screamed as loud as she could and started crying. I tried to explain the chart to her as I normally had to, but was getting nowhere.

"I'll take you into see Ms. Betsy," I stated calmly. This usually snapped her to attention, but today she kept on with her tantrum. Wanting to follow through on my word, I took her into the office to talk to my boss, Ms. Betsy, with whom she has had a very long, personal relationship. This, however, led to serious self-harm, including head banging and deep scratching. I wanted to jump in and hold her hands, and stop her from hurting herself. But I knew that I wasn't allowed to do that, especially not right in front of my boss. As we let Amy calm herself down, Betsy took me aside and mentioned that Amy had not received the adequate medication for the day because of a miscommunication between parents and the Camp Nurse. This was the first I was hearing about this, on a day where Amy had been having meltdown after meltdown. I felt instantly frustrated with my supervisors for not making me aware, especially when they had seen me struggling with her behaviors. I also then felt overwhelmed about how to handle the rest of the day with the knowledge that she had no medicine to help her.

As a camp counselor working with children with special needs, this is the line I found myself constantly straddling. Do I make exceptions for her and let her spend more time in the pool? Is this just giving in to her and teaching her that negative behavior receives positive rewards? How do I negotiate her special needs without making her stand out from all the kids there? I couldn't help but feel that if I hadn't punished her, the whole situation could have been avoided. However, I knew that if I treated her differently than I would have treated a child at camp without special needs, this would have cheated her from an opportunity to belong and a sense of inclusion. While her intellectual and social skill building happens in a different way than most children her age, I felt like not punishing her would have meant I was treating her like she had no agency for herself, which I feel perpetuates negative stereotypes about people with disabilities.

As an employee of the camp, I was angry. I felt like this was pertinent information to Amy's safety that I had every right to know so that I could offer her a safe space. My boss told me she just hadn't gotten around to finding me and telling me, but I didn't find this to be a satisfactory response. The camp administration so rigidly followed rules of confidentiality set in the organizational guidelines that necessary communication with me had not happened. They took forever to make decisions about what course of action to take in a job where quick thinking is necessary to ensure the safety of staff and campers alike. While Betsy didn't explicitly say this, I knew the administration tiptoed around sharing information regarding medication because of confidentiality procedures. However, I felt like this was a "need-to-know" situation. It was lunchtime when I found out, halfway through the day. I had spent the entire morning in the dark and was now faced with the challenge of the second half of the day with no apology from administration or explanation for the miscommunication, let alone an offer for extra support in helping Amy. While medication is not the solution to solving Amy's behavioral issues, I felt that if she wasn't using it, I should have known so that I could have been more proactive, anticipating triggers for meltdowns and ready to offer the support I knew she would need.

By the end of that day, Amy was going home and our time together was over. I felt like our session didn't end on the note it should have, given the improvement and strength in our relationship. Now, months after that incident, I still feel like a dangerous situation could have been avoided. I'm not sure what I could have done differently, but better communication was definitely needed and I still feel slightly resentful of my camp's administration for not recognizing the situation and helping me prevent it. I never approached my boss about the situation because camp had wrapped up by then and I didn't feel like opening that can of worms. However, I still feel very upset and conflicted by the situation and wish there was some type of closure to it, for Amy's sake.

Katie's reflection

Working with children with special needs is obviously a very different type of youth work than most. However, a lot of similarities emerge that one may not first realize because they're too focused on othering the child for having a disability. Just like lots of other kids, Amy had tantrums, she had likes and dislikes (especially when it came to mealtime), and she was impatient. The difference in working with Amy was that a lot of these things were uncontrollable. While she could learn mechanisms to cope with behaviors related to her disability, her brain was just wired in a different way than most children. While I grew to love her, I was constantly confronted with tough situations where I had to be able to think on my feet and be two steps ahead of her.

Amy's parents had sent her to camp because of the supportive environment it was said to provide. She had been going since a young age and, from the stories I've heard, has come a long way since the first day she stepped foot onto camp. This progress was something to be celebrated and treasured. As a child with special needs, Amy negotiates the world around her in a completely different way than most her age. The society she lives in has certain norms and attitudes towards people with disabilities, which institutionalize the way they are treated. At camp, these preexisting systems and norms are supposed to disappear. Instead of being treated differently, Amy is supposed to be treated like a normal 12-year-old girl. In our relationship, it is my responsibility as a counselor to provide that for her. I was in that job to offer a loving, supportive, and nonjudgmental atmosphere. How was I supposed to properly do this without an effective partnership between the camp administration and myself? They were supposed to guide me as much as I guided her. Without communication between us, I felt like we were failing Amy's camp experience.

In this type of setting, being able to be steps ahead of any situation is key. Some of Amy's behaviors were unpredictable, but as I learned about who she was, I was able to appraise situations and react appropriately in order to make sure she was kept safe and happy. I had to always keep in the front of my mind how to keep Amy out of risky situations and behaviors over everything else. We had weeks of orientation at the beginning of camp with trainings and briefings on procedures for different situations. This training was meant to acquaint us with our coworkers, familiarize us on camp behavioral policies and how to handle medical emergencies, and further explain our role to us. It was hard to have a two-week long orientation prepare me for an unpredictable summer, but for the most part, this orientation was able to offer me support in my actions and enabled me to negotiate situations. However, on that day I felt like they failed me.

It was hard to identify the problem initially. While Amy was known to act out from time to time, large-scale, physical meltdowns were uncharacteristic. While I tried to pay attention throughout the morning to any differences in my mood, our schedule, or anything else that could have been negatively affecting her, I didn't find anything. The only probable solution I came up with was that she was sad to be leaving later that day and couldn't express that to me. After finding out before lunch that Amy was not on her medication, I tried to go about the day as normally as possible. However, the meltdowns kept occurring at random. I did not want to separate her from the group and other activities because I knew participating was beneficial to her, but I also saw her ability to participate waning throughout the rest of the day. I didn't want to put other counselors or campers at risk, so I felt like I was in a constant battle between Amy's intrinsic needs and other people's safety. Then, I thought, how do I punish her? I know that her behaviors are not entirely her fault or under her control, but I also felt like I couldn't just let them go the rest of the day. I was constantly negotiating with my own morals in my head that day, trying to strike a balance of good cop, bad cop, with myself playing both roles.

I never did separate her from the group because I felt like that was a distinct contradiction of the camp's mission and my own beliefs. I also thought it would be detrimental to our relationship if I started depriving her of the inclusive treatment she deserved. There were so many things to consider and one correct solution never seemed to pop into my head and ring and buzz and say: "THIS ONE! THIS IS WHAT YOU SHOULD DO!" Months after the dilemma, it still hasn't become clear to me. I feel like, in terms of helping Amy, I did all I could do while staying true to how I thought she deserved to be treated. The only thing I wish I had done differently was to confront the administration. At the time, I felt like it wasn't worth the trouble on the last day of camp; but thinking about it now, Amy's needs should have been enough to get me to act on her behalf.

I had never had the strongest relationship with my administration. The core values of my camp were "spirit, honesty, wellness, and compassion." These values were supposed to be illustrated in every single action we did and word we said. However, I felt like these didn't necessarily apply to administration. If they respected Amy and me, they would have taken further precautions to ensure her wellness. They never seemed to take the counselor's side and always left us hanging without much support. It made them hard to approach with problems because you were usually left feeling even more confused than when you began. I had problems with them with other campers besides Amy. For example, one time I felt physically threatened by Matthew—my very first camper, mentioned in the introduction—and didn't feel like I could adequately serve his needs because of this. Besides being told to calm down for five minutes, my concerns were not heard or addressed. This type of power dynamic didn't breed the best relationship, and so when a particularly big issue arose, I felt like I was between a rock and a hard place.

Now it's almost been five months since that dilemma and I still think about it. If I had resolved it, maybe it would be different, but I can't help but feel like I didn't take enough action. As far as I know, Amy's just as great as always. She started middle school even! But, even if that one day didn't have a large effect in the grand scheme of things, wasn't it my job as a youth worker to make that one day count?

Unpacking the dilemma

Looking back on her dilemma with Amy, Katie is able to see the situation from both a personal viewpoint as well as an organizational one. She reflects on her inner battle to negotiate Amy's needs with her own beliefs about working with youth and how this affected the way in which she dealt with Amy's behavior on that last day of camp. Even many months later, Katie is still uncomfortable with her handling of the situation. However, what stands out more than her self-doubt about her decision-making is her disappointment in the camp administration about not sharing critical information. Katie feels that she was unable to fully identify the problem in this scenario because she was not given adequate information to assess the situation correctly. The camp's rules and procedures were upheld for the camper's privacy and safety. However, Katie's dilemma reveals where this lack of flexibility can be contradictory to the program because it put Amy, other campers, and the staff at risk by contributing to a potentially harmful situation. We now use the Ecological Dilemma Resolution model to analyze Katie's dilemma.

Knowledge

Katie acknowledges that she does not have experience working in an inclusive setting or with youth with special needs. In resolving her situation with Amy, we can see how she brings in her beliefs about equity and fairness, training received from camp, and practice-knowledge developed over the course of the summer.

Dilemma Resolution Cycle

Problem identification

Katie conveys that it was hard to identify the problem initially. Amy was known to act out but the type and frequency of physical resistance and outbursts she displayed that day were uncharacteristic. Katie ran through the morning to see if maybe there was something she was doing differently or a change in the routine that triggered Amy, but nothing stood out to her as different. Given no obvious other causes, Katie concluded that Amy was probably sad to be leaving later that day and did not have the ability to express that feeling.

Plan formulation

Katie builds her relationship with Amy based on the camp's ideals around inclusion. Katie tries to not make exceptions for Amy. Katie decides to apply the same expectations to Amy because not doing so would deny her agency and go against the camp's expectations.

Plan implementation

After Amy's multiple meltdowns, including during her morning swim, Katie decides she needs to take away part of the afternoon swim as a fair punishment for her actions. Katie uses the behavior chart to show Amy the consequence of her not listening. However, on this particular day, these approved and agreed upon sanctions did not work. In an atmosphere where Amy is supposed to be treated as a "normal 12-year-old-girl," this was a moment where her disabilities could not go unnoticed and uncared for. Katie knew this and describes how she was "constantly negotiating with my own morals in my head that day, trying to strike a balance of good cop, bad cop, with myself playing both roles." Instead of pulling Amy away from the group to do one-to-one activities, Katie follows camp policies by taking Amy to see Ms. Betsy as a form of punishment. Katie was surprised that even the threat of this action did not snap Amy out of her behaviors.

Evaluation/reflection

Upon reflection, Katie comes to see that what she was experiencing as an individual dilemma was actually an organizational tension. Upholding the confidentiality of campers' personal information is a high priority for the camp and many programs working with youth also share this commitment. However, the camp has to balance its policies on privacy with ensuring staff have the information they needed to work effectively with the youth. As we can see in this case, limited communication negatively impacts the service being given to youth. Amy's behavior put others' safety at risk and leads Amy to eventually harm herself. Without flexibility to their rule, Katie is not able to do her job to the best of her ability, which jeopardizes the emotional and physical well-being of those involved.

Katie feels like communication at the camp between staff and directors is not valued or seen as a vital component to the program culture. She does not feel supported and is given little voice in how organizational decisions are made. She questions: "How was I supposed to properly [offer a loving, supportive, and nonjudgmental atmosphere] without an effective partnership between the camp administration and myself?" She begins to see that what is best for a young person in any particular moment might directly go against organizational expectations.

REFLECTING ON PRACTICE:

What does Katie do well in this story? What strengths does she bring to youth work?

Where does Katie get stuck in this story? What keeps her from moving through the Dilemma Resolution Cycle?

Do you think Katie approached her challenges with Amy effectively? How would you have approached working with Amy?

Should the camp have notified Katie earlier about Amy's medication situation? Why or why not? When can sharing confidential information with front-line youth workers be best for the youth? The youth worker? The program?

In what ways can you relate to Katie's experience? Have you ever been in a situation in which you felt organizational policies got in the way of the work you were doing with the youth? What happened? How did you manage in that situation?

Summary

Katie's inability to assess the situation successfully was not so much due to lack of skill as it was due to incomplete information. She clearly needed help with the situation and did not receive it soon enough. The ability to ask for help is a crucial skill in all fields and something that could have benefited Katie if she had done it earlier in the day. Katie was using all her usual "tricks" with Amy but they weren't working and she knew that something with Amy's behavior was off. Still, Katie acted very much alone to solve the problem. Yes, Katie was working with Amy in an assigned one-to-one situation; however, youth development at any organization can never fully and truly be the work of one adult. When Katie did decide to go to Ms. Betsy, is was her last stop as a way to hopefully get Amy to snap out of it due to fear of getting in trouble. While administration can often play the role of dealing with behavioral issues, this should not be the only way they are perceived by staff. Going to see Ms. Betsy earlier and utilizing administration as a source of support could have brought attention to the medicine issues sooner and perhaps diffused the entire dilemma. Additionally, with more experience, Katie might have better known her own limits and abilities as a youth worker and known to seek assistance sooner.

Digging deeper: applying the dilemma to your work

Activity 1: choose an alternate scenario

Below is a list of alternate scenarios that could have arisen in the dilemma. In pairs or small groups, create a role play based on the alternate scenarios. Be sure to consider what actors are present, how each may react, and what other various ecological factors may influence the situation. After, discuss which course of action you would be most likely to take, and which you wouldn't. Explain why.

1   Counselor confronts the administration at the end of the day about why she was not informed about the medication issue earlier.
2   Counselor confronts the administration when Amy is still at camp about why she was not informed about the medication issue earlier.
3   Counselor talks to other staff about the issue and how she should approach administration.
4   Counselor does not punish Amy for not getting out of the pool.
5   Counselor separates Amy from group activities for the rest of the day and does activities one-on-one with her.

Activity 2: defining organizational support

Describe what organizational support looks and feels like to you? Is it being in complete agreement with organization administration about core values? About operating procedures? Is it feeling like the higher-ups have your back? Is it having a horizontal power structure? Is it transparent communication between all staff? Does your boss have to feel like your friend? Whatever your opinion, Katie does not feel like she had the support she needed from the Camp Directors.

In order to be proactive in understanding your organization's policies and how they may be enacted in particular dilemma situations, scan your organization's policies and answer the following:

•   What are your organization's policies about sharing information? What else did you learn about your organization's expectations by reading the policies?
•   What support systems exist at your organization/program? How and when should youth workers expect help and support from coworkers and administration?
•   Are there certain rules and/or policies that you believe should be maintained no matter what? Were there any you felt would need to be interpreted on a case-by-case basis? When can and should youth workers have autonomy in decision-making? If your beliefs may come in conflict with the formal policies, have a conversation with your supervisor so you can gain deeper understanding about how to adhere to the policies.
•   What information regarding youth should be shared with front-line youth workers?
•   What strategies do you have when asking for help? How do you assess your own skills and become comfortable with knowing where you might be limited?
•   How can asking for help not be perceived as a sign of weakness?
•   What role can coworkers play in situations where front-line staff feel unsupported by administration?

References

Dennehy, J., Gannet, E., and Robbins, R. (2006). *Setting the stage for a youth development associate credential.* Houston, TX: National Institute on Out-of-School Time for Cornerstones for Kids.

Khashu, A. and Dougherty, N. (2007). *Staffing practices of high-quality after-school programs.* Houston, TX: The After-School Corporation for Cornerstones for Kids.

8

ACTIVATING PERSONAL KNOWLEDGE TO BALANCE THE NEEDS OF HIGH-RISK YOUTH WITH THE SAFETY OF OTHERS IN THE PROGRAM

"They're just not those people when they're in our building."—Jessica

---

Chapter learning objectives

- Activating personal knowledge
- Balancing the needs of a few "high-risk" youth with the safety of the overall program population
- Disciplining youth who have violated expectations while maintaining relationships with them and keeping them connected to the program
- Using personal and professional networks to evaluate and resolve a dilemma

---

Violence that occurs outside the walls of youth development organizations can affect the job of a youth worker. One way youth workers are impacted is when they must make difficult decisions about if and how to stay connected to youth involved with violence and gangs while preserving the safety and well-being of the other young people in their programs. Youth workers need to understand why young people engage in serious violence in order to respond appropriately.

Youth workers who grew up in the same (or similar) neighborhoods as the youth they work with have access to particular types of knowledge that can be useful in resolving these situations. They have borne witness to generational cycles of violence. They understand why parents would encourage their children to use violence to settle differences (Canada, 2010). They are familiar with community resources and leaders who can help to address violence. Working with the idea that some young people grow up learning that violence is a necessary part of survival produces a number of very complex dilemmas.

At the heart of these dilemmas is whether it is possible to counter the survival skills taught at home and, if it is possible, whether youth workers can and/or should take on this incredibly difficult responsibility. How do you tell a youth that what their family is encouraging them to do is wrong, particularly when you were taught the same thing growing up? Addressing serious youth violence complicates what it means to put young people at the center of your actions when that action may be to exclude high-risk youth who are involved in serious acts of violence. These types of considerations reveal limitations of youth work and call out the larger systems that need to be involved to address youth and gang violence.

In this chapter, we tell Jessica's story. Jessica grew up in the city where she now works, and she shares many of the life experiences of the youth in the city. One recent summer, Jessica's community experienced an uptick in gang-related violence. One particularly high-profile incident occurred when Y-Block gang members stabbed two brothers at a local mall. The brothers were not in a gang, but they did live in the neighborhood of the rivaling UGE gang. The brothers survived and the perpetrators of the stabbing were apprehended by the police; however, this incident set the stage for a summer and fall of retaliatory acts of violence between Y-Block and UGE.

Jessica grew up in one of the gang-affiliated neighborhoods in the city and has family members who are in the same gangs as the young men involved in this story. She can understand why some of the young men who attend her programs resort to violence to settle differences. She can empathize with these young men's negative attitudes toward law enforcement, having her own ambivalence about working with law enforcement. However, her story differs from the young men in that she made deliberate efforts to disrupt the cycle of violence in her community. In high school, she became a peer leader and sought out mentors who could guide her analysis of the problem and help her think through ways to reach the young men. Later, when she became program staff, those around her were consistently impressed with her reliability, follow-through, and willingness to ask hard questions. Over the years, she built an impressive network of people she could turn to for information, knowledge, resources, and help. This network includes OGs (original gangsters) in her family, her mentors, her peer youth workers, and directors of the organizations whom she impressed with her work ethic. Jessica is an embedded and connected youth worker. Her reflections on what was happening with young people that summer and her own responses to those events can help us learn more about the practice of youth work in general and assist youth workers who did not grow up in neighborhoods with high levels of violence to know what to do when faced with these situations.

Jessica's story

The mall stabbing deeply affected our organization. We have satellite sites in various neighborhoods which happen to correspond to the turf of rival gangs, including Y-Block and UGE. On a day-to-day basis that summer, it felt as if members of the different sites were at war with each other. It was sad to us because it was their families and geographic locations in the city that predestined them to be lifelong enemies. We didn't see the young people as "gangsters" though, but rather as young people caught in the crossfire of a feud that began well before their time. The tensions really came home one evening during this summer when two rival gang members who were both members of our organization were involved in a non-fatal shooting. Ariel was the victim and Samuel was the perpetrator.

Ariel, a 16-year-old self-identified UGE gang member, had been involved with one of the satellite sites for about two years. He was never consistent with his attendance and came mainly to play basketball. Some of the staff described him as one of the troublemakers. He would talk back to us, disrupt games, and refuse to follow the rules. I had reached out to his parents in the past and realized that they probably would not be of any help because they were deep into the gang and drug-dealing lifestyle. Samuel was 17 years old and had been coming to our main site since he was 12. When he hit his late teenage years, he began to be more interested in the street life than what we had to offer. His grades began to drop, his school attendance was questionable, and his drive for sports fell. Samuel is affiliated with the Y-Block gang.

So going back to the evening of the shooting, it appears that Ariel was on a city bus when he noticed Samuel was also on the bus. Ariel got off the bus and realized that Samuel followed him. They had a verbal altercation and then Samuel pulled out a gun. Ariel tried to run, but he was shot in the leg. Ariel was brought to the emergency room. Later that night, in a different part of the city, UGE retaliated against Y-Block and shot a 17-year-old UGE gang member in the abdomen.

These shootings happened over a weekend and I hadn't heard about them until Monday when I came to work. I was devastated by the news. My first question was whether anybody was seriously hurt. When I found out that Ariel was in the hospital, but not with life-threatening injuries, and Samuel had been locked up, I called the Program Director to get more details on who exactly was involved in the incident.

As the news sunk in, I realized that I wasn't really shocked to hear which kids were involved, but it was still difficult to comprehend. Even though they're not the best kids, it still seemed out of character for them to be shooting at each other; it seemed like a completely different level of violence. I knew both young men quite well. Before this incident, I had been working closely with Ariel's school to get him re-enrolled after he had dropped out. As for Samuel, he had worked with us as part of the summer youth employment program. During the summer, he was a completely different person. We had no sense he would be involved in this type of incident. We vouched for him big time with the police department's Gang Unit so that he could be part of the summer youth employment program.

We went to the hospital to see how Ariel was doing and he was being discharged just as we got there. We were only able to speak to him for about two minutes before his mother told him it was time to go. Ariel assured us that he would stop by to see us later on that day. I let him know that I would need to consult with the rest of the staff to figure out the terms under which he'd be allowed to participate in programs.

We (the senior staff team) sat with the Executive Director to discuss what to do. Our primary concern was, of course, the safety of all the kids. We also discussed how this incident affected our organization's reputation and how our school and law enforcement partners would view us in light of the role some of our members played in the violence. An officer from the Gang Unit who worked closely with us was clear in his recommendation—he felt we should "boot them." The decision wasn't that easy, however. We talked about how Ariel and Samuel were very popular members at two of our outreach sites and if they stopped showing up, they might pull their friends with them. We were aware that this could affect our teen numbers and even membership totals. More importantly, however, we were cognizant that the young people most in need of a safe, supervised space may choose the streets instead to be with their friends. I also remained very worried about what was going to happen after Ariel got out of the hospital. I knew we had to prevent more acts of retaliation. I wondered if it was best to let them come back in order to keep them closer to us. Ultimately, the Executive Director's position was to ensure everyone's safety; he felt it was necessary to suspend Ariel and Samuel's membership. Later that afternoon when Ariel arrived, we told him that he would not be allowed back until he told us and showed us that he was ready to change his lifestyle.

With the immediate situation more or less under control, I reached out to people I knew in the community to find out what was going on. I knew it was important to get information on the level of tension in the gangs and how the older members saw the incidents of that weekend. I was raised in a situation that gave me access to the "thug" life, and I could ask family and friends about the incidents that took place. I had also been a peer leader in the city for a long time and had made a lot of connections with agencies. Our organization had a 15-year-plus relationship with the Gang Unit and I had worked at the Police Department's summer camp. The Gang Unit officers were impressed with work I had done at the camp, keeping things organized. Although I look really young, I get things done—so I think up until this point I had proved myself to them and they could see that we're all here for the same thing. All the work we did with the Gang Unit let me connect with those officers to discuss the possibility of further retaliation that could happen near or at our outreach sites.

After many discussions, neither the OGs nor the Gang Unit thought there was a high degree of risk for a violent act to happen near us. The Gang Unit did agree to patrol the neighborhood very closely for the next few days. I then organized Gang Awareness talks with the youth at each site. An officer from the Gang Unit went to each location and had real-life discussions with the young people. He told his own story; how as a young person he grew up in the same circumstances as them—in the projects with a single mother. He had to work hard to change his life. He told them that there are positive support systems for them and that they should keep coming to our organization.

About two months after the incident, Ariel came back to us. I arranged a meeting with his mother, other staff, and the Gang Unit. During the meeting, we noted that his mother was not supportive. At one point when Ariel was trying to explain his plans to change, she told him to shut up. But, I really felt it was obvious that he had genuine yearning to change his life. We allowed him to come back with some stipulations, including regular attendance at school and community service. For a while, he complied. He came after school, did his homework, and tried to act positively. Unfortunately and perhaps not surprisingly this was short-lived. Ariel was deeply embedded into the gang lifestyle with a family that encourages this behavior. His commitment to change his life could not compete with the draw of the streets. Within a few weeks, the Gang Unit informed us that Ariel was still actively involved with the UGE gang. We had to terminate his membership until he truly decided to change his life.

Jessica's reflection

My family is a family of seven. And my mom's from a big family. Some of my relatives are into the gang life. I've seen what violence does and what the gang life does to families firsthand. My house was raided when I was five years old. My father was involved in a drug transaction that went wrong and he was stabbed and in jail for drug-related charges for most of my early childhood. I'm sure somewhere those things come into how I think about the police and violence, so part of me can understand where the youth are coming from.

My mom at some point realized she wanted a different life for her children. She broke away, which makes the family dynamics quite interesting. There are those who are heavily involved in the gang life and those who are not. The two groups do not spend much time together. There might be a BBQ in the summer, but when we see each other, it's pretty informal. People don't talk about what they are doing and that's how we can all be together. It's a lot easier if you don't have to deal with them. But I definitely learned early on how to tell when someone is doing something they shouldn't. It's not something that I was told or taught as much as it is something I picked up.

My personality has always been to put myself around people who I think I can learn something from. I watch other people around me and what their reactions are to situations. I have had a lot of conversations with my mentors about the difference between hard-core "thugs" and the wannabe "pretty boys." So, I don't know if it's immersing yourself in the environment until it becomes instinctual for you to just react to things the way you're supposed to react. I don't know if it's naturally in you, or at some point you develop this ability. I truly believe that what I've gone through is why I am where I am now, and I think that everything that I participated in had something to do with that. But I don't think that that's the only reason I can connect with young people. I think that if you have a genuine interest in their lives and what they're doing, that's what matters.

As part of my role as coordinator of our targeted gang prevention program, I've started going to the School Department's safety protocol meetings. At these meetings, they review a list of about 100 kids in the schools that they suspect are gang involved. I've been struck and dismayed that so many of them are kids I have worked with. I just can't help but feel that they're just not those people when they're with us.

Samuel is a perfect example. He is a Hispanic kid living in a poor neighborhood, so in a sense I understand that he needs to defend himself. But to be the kid who I found out he was after the shooting? No. I just couldn't believe it. And after speaking with someone else I know who's in the gang, they say the same thing. Samuel definitely has two faces. He's very polite. All summer, he spoke professionally and was well mannered. He got along with everyone! I can't remember a single altercation involving Samuel. He was polite to the cops. He played the part really well. But the cops knew him. They told us they didn't want him. They didn't want anything to do with him. We vouched for him though. We convinced the Gang Unit that Samuel had changed. And to his credit, Samuel presented himself that way, so the police gave him the chance. And it worked out well. He made it through the whole summer. But then, about a month and a half later, he's shooting Ariel.

As I think about it, when certain expectations are set for young people, that's what they follow. If they are expected to be bad then they're going to be bad. Here, we just don't look at that. A young person comes in and we want to get to know them and what they like to do. Then we try to put them into programs and give them opportunities that reflect that. So we see the young people in terms of their potential to make their own lives. But when something like this incident happens, I always have to ask myself: "Why doesn't what we do with them last when they leave our building? How can our long-term hopes for young people actually protect them when they go back out into the streets?"

I know the answer to my own question. They go back into reality. I know that there is a sense of comfort and safety here and we become like another family for them. But when they go back into the real world and everyone is expecting them to be this other person, they just fall into it. A lot of the staff have worked here for a number of years, but the bottom line is we are not their family. Their family will be with them forever. At some point, there is a line drawn between us and them, even though I think we do a really good job of trying to be part of their lives.

Again, we can look at Samuel about how this plays out. His father has been in and out of prison. He is gang involved. So yes, Samuel can be a great kid here with us but when he goes back home, there are certain expectations that his family has of him that has become his norm. I don't know that a teenager can really articulate themselves to their parents to let them know that they want to change and want to be something other than what their parents are without shutting their parents out of their life and creating a barrier between them. I think that given the opportunity, Samuel would want a different life. But how does he then go back and explain that to his father without tarnishing their relationship? Ariel's situation was really similar. I know that with Ariel there weren't many rules set for him in the household. Then there were the rumors that his father had given him a gun to protect himself. You have to look at the whole picture. I don't know at what point we become strong enough as a youth development movement to break that kind of cycle for our participants.

Unpacking the dilemma

Three major dilemmas confronted Jessica in her handling of the aftermath of gang-related violence. The first was the enormous task of ensuring the safety and well-being of Ariel, Samuel, other participants, and neighbors of this youth organization. The second dilemma was attempting to understand the motivations of high-risk, gang-involved youth and what could encourage them to get out of the gang lifestyle. The third dilemma was more existential. Jessica struggled with the purpose of her work given the number of young people she has known who have succumbed to gang involvement. Jessica's narrative demonstrates her ecological intelligence and her application of personal and practice knowledge in the resolution of these dilemmas. In her resolution of these dilemmas, Jessica moves through the Ecological Dilemma Resolution model quite effectively.

Knowledge

Jessica's ability to persevere comes from her considerable firsthand knowledge of gang violence in the city. She has the personal knowledge to understand the dynamics of gangs and the pull of street life not because of something she read or studied but because she grew up in it. She has a deeper understanding of what the youth involved in the shootings are going through. She talked about her own experience seeing members of her family selling drugs and being arrested, and having her house raided as a child. She has longstanding connections with former gang members and police officers in the Gang Unit. She sees youth being pulled in opposite directions; trying to be one person at the outreach site and another at home or in their neighborhood. This becomes especially clear when Jessica speaks of Samuel who wants to change his life yet is thwarted in his efforts because of his fear of harming relationships with family members. Perhaps what gives Jessica hope is that she knows it is possible for individuals to choose to leave the street life; her mother consciously made this decision. Jessica herself is on a substantially different path than many of her cousins. Yet she is not naively optimistic because she knows the personal costs of making the decision to separate from family and is aware of the reality of life outside the walls of the youth organization. And so the critical question here stands: how can youth workers put their personal and practice knowledge into action to achieve an effective outcome for high-risk youth?

Dilemma Resolution Cycle

Problem identification

After the shooting between Samuel and Ariel, Jessica and the senior staff team needed to find a solution regarding the future involvement of the young men involved. Their primary concern was how to maintain the safety of Ariel and Samuel, all the youth at their various sites, and the surrounding neighborhoods.

Plan formulation

Jessica and senior staff take multiple considerations into account. They consider what is best for Samuel as an individual, Arial as an individual, and the organization as a safe place for other youth. They take the time to try to get as many voices at the table as possible and use the resources available to make sure they do not make a hasty decision.

Plan implementation

We see how Jessica was able to sift through multiple considerations quickly. She checked on the status of the victim. She deliberated with her coworkers and superiors about disciplinary and safety protocols to put into place. She consulted with OGs and police partners to assess the likelihood for retaliation. Jessica attempted to address the allure of gangs for other members by arranging for the Gang Unit to come in and hold some "real talk" sessions with the young people. These talks were not meant to scare the youth out of joining gangs, but rather to show them that there are positive alternatives available to them. Jessica is particularly effective not only because she can see and act at multiple levels in a calm and efficient manner, but also because of her considerable social capital derived from growing up in the city and in local youth organizations.

Evaluation/reflection

Some youth workers may have been tempted to give up if they had been in Jessica's shoes. Jessica had worked with Ariel and Samuel very closely. She had invested a lot of time and emotional energy in them. Beyond Ariel and Samuel, she expresses dismay at seeing so many names of youth she has worked with on the school's safety protocol list. While she recognizes that the young people are "not those people when they are with us," she also expresses her frustration at the limitation of youth work to inoculate young people from the dangers of street violence. We see this when she asks herself, "why doesn't what we do with them last when they leave our building?" and later answers her own question by acknowledging that when youth leave, "they go back to reality." This is where Jessica's dilemma becomes the most complex. She is keenly aware that gang involvement and violence are a part of these young peoples' lives as a means to survive and be accepted by their family. Therefore, she understands that their time spent with dedicated youth workers cannot necessarily change the reality of their lives outside of the building. Yet she still wonders, with a sense of perceptible hope, how the youth development movement can break these kinds of cycles and become a more powerful and positive force for the young people that need it most.

REFLECTING ON PRACTICE:

What does Jessica do well in this story? What strengths does she bring to youth work? It appears that Jessica moves effectively through the Dilemma Resolution Cycle. Do you agree? If not, where do you think she gets stuck?

What systems does Jessica consider as she comes up with her plan to try to keep the youth involved? Are there any other systems or considerations you feel she overlooked? Is there anything she did that you would not have considered? Is there anything she did that you don't agree with?

Struggling to adhere to or go against family values is a prominent theme in this dilemma. In what ways can you relate to Jessica's and the youth's struggles in this regard?

When a youth worker doesn't have personal knowledge like Jessica's, how can they still be effective? Can an 'outsider' youth worker gain the type of knowledge Jessica has?

Have you ever been faced with the decision that forced you to weigh the well-being of one youth against the well-being of other youth in your program? How did you resolve that dilemma?

What other dilemmas do you see in this case? How would you frame the problem? What types of plans would you formulate?

Summary

It is clear that Jessica's personal and practice knowledge plays a key role in how she perceives and addresses this dilemma. Jessica also uses her vast personal and professional connections to assess the situation and understand the level of risk to the youth involved as well as to other youth members. She has access to knowledge other youth workers may not have. This personal and practice knowledge allows her a deeper understanding of what the youth involved in the shooting are going through and she sees how much the two youth need a safe place like the outreach sites. Jessica's experiences fuel her motivation to make every effort to keep Ariel and Samuel connected to the organization. She can see the possibility of leaving the street life for something better, but she also is realistic and knows what she is up against.

Jessica uses a foundation of personal and practice knowledge to view the dilemma and is able to take multiple considerations into account when deciding what action to take. As she assesses the situation and develops a plan of action, Jessica keeps the youth at the center of her decision considering the needs of the youth to be supported and to be given an "out" of their violent surroundings. She balances the needs of the youth involved in the violence with the needs of the non-involved youth to have a safe place as well. She scaffolds Ariel's reintegration by holding him accountable for his actions. After thorough plan formulation, implementation, and reflection, she still must exclude Ariel from the organization. Jessica reflects on her dilemma resolution process and she is still hopeful, even though this situation ended with losing Ariel to street violence, that it is possible to draw young people away from the streets and keep them engaged in positive activities.

Digging deeper: applying the dilemma to your work

Activity 1: map your community

Jessica has an extensive network of support, knowledge, and resources in the community. What resources would you draw on in your community if confronted with this type of situation? Make a list of all community resources you have available to you. Think of both formal and informal resources. Don't forget churches, schools, and city government. Ask youth about resources they know about in the community to enhance your list. Consider mapping the resources to increase your familiarity with them and to understand how they are distributed in your city. This is especially important if you are working in a community that you are new to. Go over your list and map with coworkers and get their feedback. Develop a plan for how to build relationships with staff at other organizations.

Activity 2: activate your personal knowledge

How does Jessica's personal knowledge of the youth's environment help her navigate the situation? Revisit your autobiography, developed in Chapter 2. Reflect on your own history and how this has built your knowledge base. How could your personal knowledge (or lack thereof) be a hindrance to your youth work? If you are a community "outsider," what types of experiences do you have that could help you in situations like the one Jessica faced? Do you think that when working with high-risk youth, personal knowledge of the community in which the young people live is necessary? Why or why not?

Activity 3: involving high-risk youth

Can youth be gang-involved and still participate in your youth programs? Brainstorm safety procedures and guidelines that your program can implement and maintain, particularly when participants may be very high risk or gang involved. Refer back to Activity 1. What referral sources are available to you to better support high-risk youth?

References

Canada, G. (2010). *Fist, stick, knife, gun: A personal history of violence*. Boston: Beacon Press.

9

"WHEN I HEARD WHO IT WAS, I KNEW IT WASN'T A REAL GUN"

"Reading" the context to maintain safety[1]

Chapter learning objectives

- Being able to read potentially dangerous situations rapidly
- Using reflection as a tool to transform personal experience into practice knowledge
- Seeking out and learning from mentors

Although gun violence may seem like a rare dilemma for a youth worker to confront, we include gun dilemma stories for several reasons. First, youth gun violence is not infrequent enough in urban settings in the United States. A recent release by the Centers for Disease Control found that the rate of firearm homicides among youths aged 10–19 slightly exceeded the rate among persons of all ages in the majority of major cities. For youths aged 10–19, firearm homicide was the second leading cause of injury death (Kegler *et al.*, 2011). Second, because the stakes are so high, this type of situation reveals limitations in reliance on book knowledge and formal training in cultivating youth worker expertise. As the stories reveal, youth workers who are effective in these types of situations possess a deep understanding of the context and individuals' motivations. They are able to read a situation, not just a textbook. Finally, extreme gun violence is on a continuum with other more common forms of violence, such as fighting and gang involvement, thereby increasing the need for youth workers who can handle these types of situations.

The dilemma stories in this chapter provide in-depth examples about how youth workers draw on "personal knowledge" to resolve complex dilemmas. Jacob and Ricardo, the youth workers featured in these stories, grew up in the same or similar neighborhoods and attended the same or similar youth programs as the youth they now serve. Their early experiences provided them with a rich education in how to navigate dangerous neighborhoods, how to "code switch" when in different peer groups and settings (Anderson, 1999), and how to negotiate complex family and peer relationships that both encourage and discourage getting ahead and moving away, as well as an expanded repertoire for thinking and acting from non-family mentors at youth programs. Their stories exemplify Higgs and Titchen's (2001) understanding of expertise as the joining of theory to practice to person.

Jacob is featured in the first story. He has worked at the same youth development organization for over 15 years. Ricardo is the focus of the second story. He has worked at a local drop-in youth center for roughly six years. Jacob is African American and Ricardo is Puerto Rican. Both grew up in the city where they now work—Jacob was born there, and Ricardo has lived there since he was nine years old.

Introducing Jacob

I grew up at the Garden, a local housing project. You could walk into a hallway in the Garden and there could be anything going on. You could see two people having sex or playing craps for money. You could see smoking, drinking, snorting—it just depended on what hallway you cut through. And we were kids, so you become a product of your environment. You start to learn some of the bad things. I can remember us being 11 or 12 years old and needing money to go to the movies. We would chew gum, stick it to the bottoms of our sneakers, and run through a hallway where the big guys were playing cards and had their money on the floor. If they caught you, you knew it was going to be a tough day; but if you got away with it, you knew just not to go around that hallway for a few weeks. The good side of it was that the neighborhood was the neighborhood, and it was tight.

I attended our local Boys and Girls Club when I was growing up. For us, the Club was home, especially during the winter time. We didn't have a basketball court so the Boys Club became our spot. I went to the Club through my senior year of high school when I was named Youth of the Year. Because I was raised in the Club, a lot of those values are my values. It's a system that I've been in forever. It doesn't work for everybody, but it helped me a lot to keep me on the right path when I was growing up.

After high school, I went to college on a basketball scholarship but got hurt my first semester. I had stressed my Achilles to the point that I wasn't able to play. I came back home and had no real motivation to do anything. I worked a bunch of different jobs, all youth related.

Things changed for me when I started working as a junior camp counselor at a local agency with Bobby, an older African American staff member. He was the first one that started really filling my head with the jump shots about what youth work was all about—how to act right, how to be a professional. Bobby was real interesting because behind closed doors he would work me over: "Little boy, you better learn; you better listen—this is not a game." I think one of the biggest things that Bobby taught me was that your relationships with children give you the freedom to be the person that will say the hard things to them. Bobby was the first one who taught me that it isn't enough to get the youth to trust you. You also need to get to the point that they feel it when they let you down. And he was really good at making me feel it when I let him down. I think that was important as far as bringing me into the whole idea of what child care work and human services was going to be about.

Eventually I got the opportunity to work at a youth development organization that had several outreach sites throughout the city. I was running one of their sites in the city's largest public housing project. They called me "El Grande Negro." The majority of the kids out there were Spanish speaking and I was the big black guy. It was tough to make sure I was communicating the right message to everybody and making sure that I was doing the right thing. By the end, the relationships that were built were solid. The kids loved me and parents that couldn't speak a lick of English trusted me. They would get their few Spanish words they knew I'd understand—"Gracias Jacob," that was it—but they knew their kids were safe with me and their kids trusted me. Now I'm the Director of Operations for this multi-site organization that serves close to 1,000 youth a year in three of the most distressed neighborhoods in the city.

Jacob's dilemma

Early one spring evening, back on what would've seemed a pretty average night, the gym was full but the rest of the building was relatively empty. The boxing gym was also packed but that was deep in the basement. There were a few random pockets of kids throughout the rest of the building. A couple hours before closing, a "part-time" member—John—showed up and started getting the guys in the gym worked up. I eased my way over to find out what was going on and found out that John was coming to "rally up some troops" because he needed backup. He told the guys inside that he was being followed by two Gangbangers and he needed to show them he had numbers backing him up, hoping to intimidate the Gangbangers to leave him alone.

My first action was to step in and tell the guys playing basketball that if they went outside and got involved in the fight then they would not be allowed back inside. Some listened and stayed inside, but others had already slipped outside with John. By the time I got to the outside steps, the two gang members were across the street; one was on a cell phone while the other was yelling at John.

Now John is the "perfect victim." He is a trash-talking loner. He doesn't have a crew or a gang backing him. He also is not someone that a whole bunch of people would be concerned about. If gang members hurt John, their personal reputations grow with little or no negative consequences for them. No one will retaliate on John's behalf, and therein lays John's value. Second, the reason why the gang members haven't attacked him yet is because they think that all these basketball players out here may jump in on John's behalf. This is why one of the guys is on a phone; he's calling for backup. Third, I realized that the gang members were up to something. I knew their faces because they've been here boxing, but they weren't talking to me; they didn't want anything to do with me. But they knew who I was. And I knew they were packing something because they were wearing large coats while it was about 60 degrees fahrenheit outside.

I thought about calling the police, shutting down the building, and calling parents to come pick up their kids. But I felt like that was an extreme reaction. I believed that if I could get all "my" guys and John back inside then the issue would die out. I knew the guys would rather finish their basketball game than get involved in John's fight. I told them: "Everybody inside if you're staying; otherwise it's time for you to go." I knew the kids would think, "I'm not missing my basketball game," and the majority of them did go back in. I also got John to come inside. The night reached cleanup time with no further incidents.

But then, as we were getting ready to close the building for the night, three older males came in looking for John. I just happened to be talking with John about what had happened that night. I immediately recognized one of the guys, Juan, as a former boxer in our program. I asked Juan why he was bringing "drama" here to us. Juan said that he did not like John and he wanted to hurt him. I could tell that tension was growing so I told all three that they had to leave since they were not members. The oldest of the three looked me in the face; he pulled up his sweatshirt just enough to show me that he had an automatic hand gun stashed in his waistband. He replied to my request with a defiant "I ain't goin' nowhere!" I replied to Juan with "here's the deal—you're not going to leave here with him; and I would suggest that you leave here with that gun because this is the wrong place for you to put yourself in this situation." He replied, "naw, man, we're takin' him."

I had thoughts of trying to blast the "gunman's" head clean off, but realized that the hallway was full of staff and youth who had begun to assemble to watch what was going down. I knew I had Chico behind me—a part-time staff person whose head was still pretty wrapped up in the street life—who had an attitude of violence begets violence. I knew I had to keep Chico out of it so that the situation would not escalate. That moment could've been life-threatening for so many people, which is why I calmed down and regained rational thought in seconds. I focused my attention on Juan, the gangbanger I recognized. I said: "We can make this real clear. Y'all take your crew and you can go. I keep John and we all leave it for tonight."

Juan made a comment to the other two: "Yo, he's cool; we don't need to have this problem with him." At that point they walked out. I followed them to the door and watched them disappear around the corner. I started to call the police to report the incident. Before I could even get the call out, a beat officer stopped in on his regular route. After hearing what happened, the officer called for backup. They were able to apprehend the two younger gang members, but not the three older ones. As it turned out, one of the younger ones had a machete and the other one had a hatchet and they both had plans to do damage.

Being in multiple potentially violent situations and situations that did get violent, you almost start to get a picture of how people react and how they're going to move. I mean you can almost look in the person's eyes and tell. There's a certain look; it's tough to explain because it's so natural—you just know if the kid has it or not. Bobby used to say all the time, "there's a switch in them." And not everybody has that switch, especially not the young guys. That switch comes through time. And you can see when that switch is hit because there is no turning back. There's a different animal coming in. A lot of people like to think the guy to worry about is the one who's jumping up and wild. Bobby taught me that that's the guy who wants you to break up the fight before it happens—that's why he's putting on a show. Bobby said that the real guy you've got to watch is the guy who moves in silence. The one who's deliberate with his movements, the one who's not taking his eyes off his focus. Those are the guys you've got to pay attention to because those are the guys that are really going to set it off.

The decisions I made that night were largely because I knew John hadn't had his switch flipped and I also knew Juan's switch has been flipped long ago. Luckily it all turned out good for my kids.

Introducing Ricardo

I'm 31 now and have been in the youth work field since I was about 16. I was born in Puerto Rico and came to the US when I was nine. After a year in another city, I moved here because my mom and the man who was in her life weren't getting along. We had to leave immediately, pack whatever we could, and come here. At first we stayed in a shelter. Eventually, my mom went back to school, got a job, and got us an apartment.

I started going to our local YMCA to play basketball when I was about 14. My neighborhood was one of the tougher ones in the city and my mom was really struggling, having to work a lot of hours to keep the family going. Going to the Y gave me a break from having to see how much my mom had to bust her butt. It gave me a mental break from having to watch where I was walking, what neighborhood I was in, and what kids I would run into. At the Y, I was all set. There were adults. I could play basketball till like ten at night. I could go home and go to bed and not have to worry about anything.

Even though I had the Y, I still did some stupid stuff as a kid. We would steal cars and go joyriding. I had a bunch of friends who sold drugs and carried guns and sometimes it was like the Fourth of July, kids would just let off shots. Kids in my group of friends would put razors in their mouths so that they could get the weapon into school and not get caught if they got searched. But if they got into a fight, they would pull that out and slice you up.

But the YMCA was good for me. I learned a lot about youth work from Martin, a staff person I looked up to. He was cool, had a lot of friends, and seemed to be living the good life. What I learned from Martin had less to do with anything he directly taught me and had more to do with what I started to realize about street life after Martin was arrested for dealing drugs. When Martin was locked up, I wrote to him. He would write back and be like, "you're the only person writing to me." And that made me realize stuff about the streets. All these people say they're your friends when you're making money and going clubbing. But none of them visited him or sent him anything when he was locked up. Me and his girlfriend were the only two people that communicated with him—not even his family.

I realized that I needed to change some things about my own life. I saw my friends graduating from selling weed to cocaine. They broke into houses to rob them. It got really messy. They would invite me every now and then. You know like, "wanna make some money?" It was tempting, but by that time I was in my late teens and had already started working with youth. I would think about Martin and how if I got caught and arrested, those so-called friends would drop me. Why would I do something that isn't going to show me love back? Especially when I have these little kids that are looking up to me now? As I got older, that became so much more important—what the youth thought versus what my friends thought—especially when I started going to school.

Taking the high road was a struggle. A lot of my friends thought I was a cornball for choosing work and school over them. They told me I was wasting my time. A lot of times it did drag me down. Eventually, I was able to get over it and complete my college degree in human services.

Ricardo's dilemma

In the mornings, when young people are not at the drop-in center where I work, I'm usually in my office, responding to emails and filling out paperwork. When the youth are on-site, I like to sit and play cards with them. Laughter and "trash" talk generally dominate our conversations. This is the space where I earn young people's trust.

Not too long ago, I dealt with something that I have never had to deal with. The day started like any other. It was starting to change over from fall to winter and this was one of the first really cold days of the season. I came in with my coffee and said good morning to the staff at the front desk. I looked inside our GED classroom and there were a good number of students listening and getting their work done. I sat at my desk and started to check my emails. I was interrupted by a couple of phone calls and when I was off the phone, Nicki, the GED teacher, approached me looking a bit nervous. My first instinct told me that maybe something personal was going on and she needed to leave early. However, as Nicki began to speak, I realized that the problem was here and now. She told me that Lisa, one of her students, came into her office during a break and expressed that she was very scared and wanted to go home. When asked why, Lisa broke down and told her that while she (Nicki) had stepped out to answer a phone call, two students started talking about some altercations they had been in in the last couple of weeks. Anthony, one of the young men, said that he didn't feel safe so he had to do something about it. Lisa pretended to not be looking but out of the corner of her eye she saw that Anthony had a gun tucked under his shirt.

This was a situation that we never had to deal with before. We had no protocol or prior experience to inform our decision-making process. First, I ran it by the

Executive Director. Initially, we thought we should call the police because we did not think we should handle such a significant safety issue on our own. Yet after considering who the youth was and the relationship we had with him, we decided not to call the police. I knew that Anthony wouldn't be a kid that would be pulling out the gun to shoot me. He's a tough kid; he's gone through stuff. I don't know how I knew, but I just did. I've been around some pretty crazy people, and he just didn't come off as one of those people. He had been coming to GED; he had a kid on the way. He was trying to do the right thing. I thought he is probably scared. I thought it was probably not even a real gun and if it was a real gun, I thought it might not even be loaded. I thought that he's probably trying to prevent people from beating him up—versus the "I want to go hurt somebody." And I thought about him bringing it to a place like this; it was more about him getting home or getting here versus him thinking "I'm looking for somebody, and wherever I see him, I'm going to shoot him." I didn't think that this is a kid who's going to hurt somebody here. He loves this place, you know? He loves the staff here. If it was a kid I didn't know then I might not have had that go through my head.

The other staff and I decided to pull Anthony into another room rather than call the police. I was quiet at first, but then I started talking. I wasn't sure what to say but I found myself telling Anthony: "You know, some students have left; we think maybe because they saw the gun. Several people say that they saw a gun on you—is this true?" Anthony admitted it. He said it was a BB gun. I told him, "I'll believe it when I see it." Anthony handed it over to the Executive Director, and she gave it to me. It did look like a gun. He had taken the safety off—the orange part that makes it noticeable that it was not a real gun. When I held it, I knew by the weight that it wasn't a real gun. While I started to breathe easier again, I knew that because he took the safety off, it would have been considered a concealed weapon. All three of us took turns talking about how dangerous it is to carry a gun. We discussed how to be safe without carrying a weapon. We also talked about the implications of carrying a concealed weapon for a youth with a criminal background.

During this conversation, Anthony expressed a deep sadness for having lost his cousin to violence very recently. He also admitted that he was having trouble with some gang members in his neighborhood. We wrapped up by saying that we would give the gun back and not alert police this time, but next time our hands would be tied and we would be forced to call. We also connected him with a mental health counselor.

After sending Anthony back to class, I called his mother. She confirmed the loss of his cousin and apologized for what he had put the staff through. We asked that she come and get him because he was still was carrying the BB gun. She couldn't get him so we called his advocate—a licensed social worker with a longstanding relationship with the center—and we released him into her protection while she brought him home.

We always will approach these situations carefully, and it's better to find out what's going on than it is to jump to conclusions. If we had called the cops, we could have easily solved the problem or we could have exacerbated the issue. If the gun was real, someone could have been hurt upon police arrival. Since the gun wasn't real, we could have sent a youth to prison for an issue we could have resolved internally. We could have sent him on his way with the BB gun, but if somebody was going to beat him up and he pulled that out and they had a real gun, then what? However, the question is are you putting yourself and others in serious danger? The relationships you have with your youth determine the kind of actions you will take when they make a mistake. Your instincts sort of take over. I am thankful that the humanitarian in us allowed us to make the right decision.

Unpacking the dilemma

A professionally educated workforce is critical for the success of youth development programs (Astroth et al., 2004; Fusco, 2011; Mattingly et al., 2002). Youth workers with knowledge about stages of child and adolescent development, theories of positive youth development, group dynamics, and program management are critical to fulfilling the mission of youth development organizations. Yet the knowledge that proved to be essential in these stories did not come from classes or textbooks. Ricardo and Jacob were able to transform their personal knowledge into actionable practice knowledge. Reading and analyzing their stories allows youth workers who have not had similar experiences insights into how to approach such dilemmas.

Knowledge

In the face of potential gun violence, Jacob and Ricardo remained calm and were able to read complex settings, events, and personalities. They formulated and enacted plans that successfully balanced the interests of the individuals holding weapons and instigating violence with the safety and well-being of the groups of youth and staff at their organizations. Jacob and Ricardo were not just lucky in their decision-making. Rather, their effectiveness was derived from a synthesis of years of experience on the job and their experiences in neighborhood peer groups and youth programs.

Jacob and Ricardo grew up in distressed, urban neighborhoods. They engaged in a range of activities with their peers, some of which were illegal and risky. Being a part of peer groups was also part of their strategy to maintain their safety as they traveled throughout the city. In so doing, they developed the capability to read situations and people, and to know who and where to avoid and how to avoid them; and ultimately they developed the ability to evade serious trouble. As teenagers, attending the Boys and Girls Club and the Y was an important part of their strategy to avoid getting into trouble and to stay safe. Over time, through formal and informal contact with staff, they further developed their ability to read situations and people, and they also acquired an expanded repertoire of beliefs and ways to act from their involvement with mentors in youth development activities. As both entered late adolescence and early adulthood, youth development organizations provided them with the opportunity to apprentice with expert youth workers.

Yet, their stories also reveal that youth workers who grow up in these neighborhoods and participate in youth programs are not guaranteed to have the type of actionable knowledge that both Jacob and Ricardo possess. For example, part of Jacob's calculation involved how to keep Chico—a staff person with "his head still too much in the street"—away from the situation. Likewise, Ricardo learned that "street credibility" was not sufficient to be an effective youth worker when one of the staff he most looked up to, Martin, got arrested for drug dealing. Chico and Martin illustrate that coming from a similar socioeconomic background as the youth and having experience in youth development programs does not guarantee youth worker expertise.

Jacob and Ricardo, on the other hand, demonstrate ecological intelligence (Walker and Larson, 2012). They both had a keen ability to see the complexity and ecological layers of problems. In Jacob's case, he was able to prioritize the safety of the youth and the organization over the need to retaliate over an act of disrespect. For Ricardo, his involvement at the Y showed him how to channel his sense of justice and deep concern for the well-being of all youth—regardless of their background or involvement in illegal activities—in a way that guided his decision to not call the police to handle the threat of gun violence. An aspect of these youth workers' expertise lies in their ability to make decisions when confronted with conflicting rules of youth organizations and the streets. Urban youth worker expertise can be explained in part by the extent to which they are able to integrate personal knowledge about the rules and practices of the streets with the values, expectations, and policies of youth organizations.

Dilemma Resolution Cycle

Problem identification

Both Jacob and Ricardo have swift and successful reactions to very complex and potentially dangerous situations. Jacob's assessment of the situation is focused on keeping the conflict from escalating. He is dealing with circumstances in which the individuals involved intend to harm a youth under his care.

Ricardo has the opposite problem in which his youth is a potential "aggressor." He uses his knowledge about Anthony to determine that he means no harm to anyone at the center; however, he recognizes that Anthony's possession of a gun inadvertently creates a safety issue for Anthony and other youth in the program.

Plan formulation

From Jacob's account, we get a clear picture of the process he used to resolve this extremely complex problem. He assessed the situation—taking into account what he knew about John and the behavior of the two younger gang members. He decided on a course of action to get "his guys" back into the Club and to process the situation with John.

Ricardo also reads a very complex situation efficiently and successfully. His analysis of the situation suggests that if they had called the police then the situation could have come out much worse for all involved. His relationship with Anthony and his ability to read him allows him to understand that Anthony was trying to maintain his own safety; he was not looking to harm anyone. Ricardo decides that the best course of action is to get Anthony in a separate room and learn why he is feeling the need to carry a gun.

Plan implementation

Jacob enacted his plan with no further incident until a group of older gang members came looking for John. At this point, Jacob realized that the three older individuals meant serious business—by their faces and the deliberateness of their actions, he knew their "switch" had been turned on. Jacob saw that he had to ensure that the rules of the "street" did not penetrate the operations of the organization. He was able to remain calm and his analysis of the situation allowed him to resolve the situation peacefully for the youth and staff. By involving the police when he did, he was able to partially resolve the illegality of the weapon activity. Jacob's integration of knowledge derived from growing up in a tough neighborhood; and having Bobby as a mentor allowed him to read the youth and the situation and to act in a way that maintained the safety of the potential victim, perpetrators, and witnesses.

Ricardo also was able to implement his plan. Although he admitted he was unsure about what he was going to say initially, once he found his words, he was able to use the relationship he had with Anthony to learn about why he was carrying the gun. Interestingly, Ricardo also learned that the assumptions he had made about the gun were accurate (i.e. that it wasn't real and that Anthony did not intend to use it on anyone at the drop-in center).

Evaluation/reflection

The gun stories illustrate two ways that reflection leads to improved youth work practice. First, reflection deepens understanding of personal beliefs, values, and motivations to engage with young people (Cusick, 2001; Fusco, 2012; Krueger, 1997). Ricardo illustrated this when he said the reason he resisted his friends' pull toward street life was because he realized that the fulfillment he got from youth work far surpassed the short-term benefits of engaging in illegal activity. Likewise, Jacob explicitly talks about how his childhood participation at the Boys and Girls Club led him to internalize the Club's values as his own, which acted as a counterbalance to lessons he learned on the street.

Second, Ricardo's and Jacob's stories show the rich knowledge they acquired over their nonprofessional lifetime about youth's motivations to engage in violence. Reflection transformed these experiences into actionable knowledge that allowed them to resolve the gun dilemmas effectively. While the idea that reflection improves practice is not new, the insights from the narratives suggest that limiting reflection to professional practice only could restrict the sharing of personal knowledge that youth workers like Jacob and Ricardo hold. As Hildreth and VeLure Roholt have discussed, youth workers need to "master a better understanding of their own biographies" (2013: 154)—both to improve individual practice and to advance the profession with the contextual theories of youth workers.

REFLECTING ON PRACTICE:

What do Jacob and Ricardo do well in their stories? What strengths do they bring to youth work? Where do they get stuck in the Dilemma Resolution Cycle?

What considerations do Jacob and Ricardo balance as they assess their situations? What were some other possible options available to Jacob and Ricardo?

Does your organization have policies about weapons? If so, do the policies allow for a youth worker to use discretion to resolve the problem? If not, do you think weapon policies should lay out clear instructions or allow for some discretion? Why or why not?

How does personal knowledge help Jacob and Ricardo to formulate a plan of action? In what way may personal knowledge be a hindrance to youth workers who face similar situations?

Consider your own history and unique knowledge base. How does this influence your work with youth? How can you access your personal knowledge more effectively?

For youth workers you supervise, how does this case make you think about mentorship differently? How can you facilitate mentorship for some of your youth workers that have grown up in similar situations to the youth they now serve?

Digging deeper: applying the dilemma to your work

Activity 1: revisit your autobiography to activate personal and practice knowledge

Go back to your youth work autobiography, developed in Chapter 2.

- What personal beliefs, values, and motivations to engage with young people does your autobiography reveal?
- What personal knowledge do you have that can be/has been turned into practice knowledge?
- Are you working with or do you want to work with young people that share similar personal knowledge and/or come from a similar background as you?

- When can it be beneficial to share a knowledge base with youth? What can make having this commonality difficult?
- When can it be beneficial to not share a knowledge base with youth?

Activity 2: reading a situation and decision-making

Think of a time when you had to make a decision in a split second in order to immediately handle a situation.

- What was the situation? Describe the key players, place, time, relevant organizational policies, etc.
- What decision did you have to make? What considerations did you have to balance to make this decision?
- Did you have support from other youth workers?
- Did you have to report anything to your organization or elsewhere after?
- Were you satisfied with your decision?
- Would you have done anything differently?

Note

1   This chapter is adapted from Ross (2013).

References

Anderson, E. (1999). *Code of the streets: Decency, violence and the moral life of the inner city.* New York: W. W. Norton & Company.

Astroth, K., Garza, P., and Taylor, B. (2004). Getting down to business: Defining competencies for entry-level youth workers. *New Directions for Youth Development, 104,* 25–37.

Cusick, A. (2001). Personal frames of reference in professional practice. In J. Higgs and A. Titchen (Eds.), *Practice knowledge and expertise in the health professions.* Oxford: Butterworth-Heinemann (pp. 91–5).

Fusco, D. (2011). On becoming an academic profession. In D. Fusco (Ed.), *Advancing youth work: Current trends, critical questions.* New York: Routledge (pp. 111–26).

Fusco, D. (2012) Use of self in the context of youth work. *Child & Youth Services, 33*(1), 33–45.

Higgs, J. and Titchen, A. (Eds.). (2001). *Practice knowledge and expertise in the health professions.* Oxford: Butterworth-Heinemann.

Hildreth, R. and VeLure Roholt, R. (2013). Teaching and training civic youth workers: Creating spaces for reciprocal civic and youth development. In R. VeLure Roholt, M. Baizerman, and R. Hildreth (Eds.), *Civic youth work: Co-creating democratic youth spaces.* Chicago: Lyceum Books (pp. 151–9).

Kegler, S., Annest, J., Kresnow, M., and Mercy, J. (2011). Violence-related firearm deaths among residents of metropolitan areas and cities: United States, 2006–2007. *Centers for Disease Control, Morbidity and Mortality Weekly Report, 60*(18): 573–8. Available at: www.cdc.gov/mmwr/preview/mmwrhtml/mm6018a1.htm (accessed January 24, 2015).

Krueger, M. (1997). Using self, story, and intuition to understand child and youth care work. *Child & Youth Care Forum, 26*(3), 153–61.

Mattingly, M., Stuart, C., and VanderVen, K. (2002). North American Certification Project (NACP) competencies for professional child and youth work practitioners. *Journal of Child and Youth Care Work, 17,* 16–49.

Ross, L. (2013). Urban youth workers' use of "personal knowledge" in resolving complex dilemmas of practice. *Child & Youth Services, 34*(3), 267–89.

Walker, K. and Larson, R. (2012). Youth worker reasoning about dilemmas encountered in practice: Expert-novice differences. *Journal of Youth Development, 7*(1), 5–23.

10

"DO THEY THINK WE'RE NOT IN CHARGE?"

Addressing dilemmas that arise in a Social Justice Youth Development approach

> **Chapter learning objectives**
>
> - Being proactive in negotiating relationships with partner organizations
> - Channeling anger and frustration into creating teachable moments for youth
> - Engaging youth in problem-solving

Youth workers operating within a Social Justice Youth Development (SJYD) framework encounter the same dilemmas as other youth workers. However, these youth workers also routinely face situations that may not be considered a dilemma if they were doing more "traditional" youth work due to SJYD's intentional focus on hierarchical power and systemic oppression (Ginwright and Cammarota, 2002). This chapter delves into such a dilemma that Colin faced while working in an urban-based SJYD group called Youth in Action (YIA).

YIA engages in environmental and food justice in a neighborhood that is comprised primarily of low-income people of color. YIA youth largely come from the neighborhood they are working in. YIA's structure is based on a worker cooperative model in which all youth and adults are staff members of equal standing and authority. All major decisions are made by youth and adults through consensus. YIA has a weekly session called "Batzaar" in which youth and adults discuss challenges and tensions during the week of work. This space of "straight talk" is often where dilemmas, internal and external, are discussed and solutions are proposed.

SJYD emerged as both a critique and expansion of traditional Positive Youth Development (PYD) (Ginwright and Cammarota, 2002). Like PYD, SJYD promotes skill development, supportive environments, and positive programming.

However, adherents of SJYD claim that PYD does not go far enough as it only focuses on individual betterment and not on the community conditions that underlie youth problems. Alternatively, SJYD connects youth issues to larger community dynamics and broader systemic power dynamics. This framework understands youth as embedded within larger changing political, economic, and social terrains, which they must navigate despite the oppression of their identities and circumscriptions to their agency. SJYD programming develops young people's critical consciousness and supports youth-led social action aimed at healing not only themselves but also the community. In SJYD, equitable youth-adult power dynamics are paramount as is democratic control over decision-making (to the degree that youth feel comfortable). Adults cannot simply decide the solutions to all dilemmas; they often must work with youth to come to an agreeable collective decision.

Introducing Colin

Colin is in his early twenties. He first became interested in doing youth work because of his own experiences as a young person. Colin grew up in a wealthy white suburb in which the needs of youth had been largely ignored. In his words:

> In my small suburban town there was nothing to do for teenagers once they hit 12—so mostly kids immediately jumped into drinking and doing whatever drugs they could get their hands on. In the four years I was in high school, there were five deaths from alcohol. This is a tiny town and I had still been close to some of these people up till the year before they died. I had addicts in my family—addiction is in my genes. I looked at my family and I saw so many of my friends fading fast down that same well-trodden path a small group of us wanted to escape.

Colin began meeting with a group of friends after school. They established a youth-run group that sought to create a youth culture that rejected drugs and alcohol, was based in direct democracy, and offered youth the opportunity to create their own support systems and activities from the ground up. The group was a success and soon began attracting young people from around the state. The group lasted five years and left Colin with a deep belief in youth empowerment, social justice, and direct democracy.

In college, Colin studied community and youth development and, starting with an internship, he fell into a long-term position at YIA as an Adult Coordinator. Colin comments on his evolution to YIA staff:

> This funny thing that I was part of when I was 14 kind of saturated my world view. At some point in college I realized my experiences as a teenager weren't just a weird fluke. I didn't know what self-determination was when I was a kid but as I tried to make sense of my world in college, I realized

these ideas were so central to movements for justice. Young people given a bit of self-determination will come up with the most creative solutions to the problems they face in the community.

He was drawn strongly towards YIA as a youth-run model that aimed to bring SJYD, cooperative values, and environmental justice together. "Who knew you could get a job like that?"

YIA's office is based in the teen center within the Draconi Towers housing project, where they have worked with residents on food justice projects both in collaboration with and in opposition to the Draconi managers. The location of YIA's office is important because the battles between the YIA youth and Draconi management are at the heart of this chapter's dilemmas. YIA was located in Draconi Towers as part of an agreement with the primary funder, a nearby university. The following dilemmas occurred while Colin was still working with YIA as an intern under a much more experienced youth worker, Kim.

Colin's dilemma

One of the youth staff—Lanh—asked Kim if he could get a key to the YIA office door so he could get to the office early to work on grant writing. Lahn, one of two founding youth members of the co-op, had shown total devotion to the program and had been essential to YIA funding efforts and communications. Knowing that YIA was facing a cash crunch, Lahn had taken on more hours to work on grant writing.

Kim asked Lanh to make his official request in Batzaar. While some of the other youth grumbled at their own need for a key, in the end it was clear that having the key implied Lahn was keen to do some extra unpaid labor, which none of the other youth were too enthused about doing. The other youth acknowledged Lahn's three years' worth of being more reliable and punctual than any of the staff, including either me or Kim. Having reached consensus in Batzaar, Kim and Lahn went to the Draconi Towers managers to see about getting a new key made for Lahn. However, the managers refused to consider the possibility on the grounds that Lahn was under 18 and the key would give him access not only to the YIA office but also to the larger Teen Center. Worried that Lahn would abuse the space if given unchaperoned access, they denied the key.

Kim and Lahn brought the issue to a Batzaar at which we decided that they could best win the key by demonstrating we were the exact opposite of Draconi management's assumptions. Kim and I both had enough community organizing experience to know that an appeal to power is the first step in negotiations before escalating to more open hostility. Knowing adultism concedes more easily to respectability than to immediate attack, we prepared a PowerPoint presentation on YIA's mission, projects, structure, and the importance of having access to our office both in terms of practicality and philosophy. Our basic strategy was to be nice, polite youngsters who appeal to their authority. We sought to break their stereotypical image of teens. We thought that they might just grant us the key if we could convince them about how responsible Lahn is and how we, as the adults, were willing to take ultimate responsibility. We knew that we were undermining the egalitarian power structure of YIA and that the approach of promoting the credibility of the work and the "articulate" young people routine is somewhat patronizing. But, we also knew that management would likely feel good about having the request made in a more formal and traditional way. We decided that particular tradeoff was worth the potential benefit of Lahn getting the key.

We set up a meeting between Draconi managers, Lahn, and Kim at which the two would give their appeal and presentation. The presentation was successful in showing that YIA was accountable and that Lahn was a responsible young person trying to do his job. A sympathetic official made Lahn a key. While we were able to resolve this dilemma successfully over the summer, by the fall Lahn had transitioned out of the group and new conflicts between YIA and management arose.

YIA's office is located in the Draconi Towers Teen Zone, which offers programs and a drop-in center to the housing project's youth. At the start of the summer, the Teen Zone had been newly renovated and stocked with a new TV, video games, a pool table, and other equipment. YIA had long had its office in the Teen Center, and worked amiably with the Center's Director; but this summer, a new director— Maggy—had been hired. YIA had immediately come into conflict with Maggy over space issues.

This conflict came to a head one evening when youth staff were working in the office late, while Kim and I were elsewhere. The Teen Zone was closing and as Maggy was getting ready to lock the doors and leave work, when she noticed that the light in the YIA office was on. She went to go investigate—knocking and opening the door to see three youth all working on various projects for the co-op, but no adult supervision in sight. Maggy told the youth that she was heading out and that they would have to leave the office because she can't leave "kids" in the Teen Zone alone. The youth were taken by surprise considering this hadn't been a problem for all of the months YIA had stayed working in the office despite the Teen Zone closing an hour earlier. The youth later reported thinking: "Why now? How can she suddenly decide to not trust us?" The youth staff put up a few counter arguments such as "but Kim is going to be back" or "but we need to get this done before we go home today." To all of their grumbling, Maggy said: "Listen, unless Kim or Colin is actually physically here, I can't let you guys stay here; it's the rules and I don't make them up." The youth complained but were eventually kicked out of the office.

The youth were furious! At our next Batzaar, they roared their complaints about Maggy's sudden assumption that YIA youth couldn't be left alone in the Teen Zone: "She must think we'll steal all the computers." "Why would we want any of that stuff? We have four computers right here!" "We should go on strike!" "Doesn't she know us?" Kim and I were angry, but less angry than the youth. I figured we'd iron this out with the same strategy of appeal to reason and being polite. I was annoyed but adultism is part of dealing with … adults. I spent a lot of time suggesting this or swearing about it with youth. But they took it to heart. It became agenda item number one. The youth decided to have another diplomatic-style meeting with Maggy to address the issue. The previous presentations on the YIA mission and cooperative ideas on youth power had worked surprisingly well, so the group agreed to repeat this approach. Kim said: "You know, if we really show them that we want this and that we are responsible workers and members of the community, maybe they'll see us differently. I think this sort of meeting will help us like it did over the summer; but unlike last time, we should really try to get Maggy to see that we aren't just here to hang out in the Zone—that we're here because it's our job." I thought this was a reasonable approach—especially since it had worked in the past.

Before we could organize the meeting with Maggy and management, Maggy kicked youth out of the office a handful of times more. At one point, she kicked out Andy who protested: "But I'm 18! That's an adult! How can you say there isn't an adult here? This is our job; I get paid for it." Maggy was apparently unsympathetic to the legal definition of adult. At this point, I began to get really pissed off at Maggy because now it wasn't about arbitrary rules but really just discriminatory nonsense. Andy was 18—three years younger than me. She was shutting him out because he was a young man of color living in the projects, not because he wasn't of age. Guilty before proven innocent. My anger was building but Kim was so much more level-headed than me. Her strategy was always to smile and nod, and then just go ahead and do whatever you wanted. "Better to apologize than to ask permission." Still I had no good solutions.

The meeting with Maggy did eventually happen, with youth striving to explain the numerous reasons that they needed to stay in their office. Topics included that she was preventing them from getting their work done, that they were staff members and were not just in the Teen Zone to hang out, that Andy is old enough to be a legal adult, and that the entire idea of adult supervision clashes with youth as bosses on equal footing with adults. Maggy overall seemed unimpressed and held firm that she was responsible for the Teen Zone and that meant when an adult was not there, no one could be. From then, either me or Kim always were to be present after hours.

The following workday, the board in our office was covered in notes of frustrations. The youth were swearing, angrily debating "what next?" The group agreed to try another meeting, this time between YIA, a handful of Maggy's superiors, and Maggy. This meeting had less youth involvement as the group began to believe that Maggy just refused to accept solutions spearheaded by youth. This too ended in non-committal solutions and eventually the same result: adult supervision is required.

It became clear that no one in YIA knew what to do. We had lost and seemingly hit a brick wall of non-discussion from Maggy. Victor remarked, "do they think that we're not in charge?" Luz responded: "Seems so, since she called us 'kids'. I'm not a kid … I'm not a kid. I'm my Mom's kid. At work I am not a kid. I'm a citizen." Victor added: "Yeah, I'm not a kid even though I'm short. We work here too."

It was at this point that I realized that this was not just going to be an inconvenience or a "teachable moment." The situation was deteriorating and the mission of YIA was going down with it. If we followed the rules, I would be babysitting them twice a week—utterly destroying any pretense of our principles of equal bosses. For Andy and Jake, it was a loss of pride. For Victor, the idea of youth–adult equality was the whole point. Victor usually stayed in the office working far later than the rest of us, always excited to be involved. For Victor, YIA was more than a job, and he took our ideals deeply to heart. It was a crushing defeat for him that he would no longer be able to work late.

That same day, we discovered that Draconi management had taken away our wireless internet modem leaving a note that said: "You cannot use your wireless router anymore as it is causing interference in the Draconi network; you can use one cable only as long as you don't touch anything else." Effectively, Draconi Towers had stolen our internet and we were only able to use the internet on one computer at a time, rendering our workday pointless.

It felt like a nightmare. All of us felt dejected, violated, and thoroughly at a loss. What was next? What could we do? With each new solution we gave up more and more SJYD values. Everywhere we resorted to authority figures. After a few weeks of youth tangling with Draconi, we had to get Kim to get the router from management. We had Alan, the YIA Director, meet with Maggy's boss in management with no results. There was nothing else to do. Our dim glimmer of resistance occurred when Victor directly disobeyed the sticky note commanding us to use only one internet jack. "I gotta get stuff done."

Colin's reflection

Looking back on this dilemma with Draconi, I see a few things we should have done. For so much of that year, I was really just following Kim's lead and was still foggy on how youth work works—all my experience was from actually being a teenager. I could have talked much more with the group to brainstorm solutions instead of just being angry. I wanted the youth to come up with something. They followed Kim's suggestion to be smart, persuasive, and polite. But when it didn't work and everyone kept getting kicked out, we just started losing steam. We couldn't get our work done; we couldn't follow our own principles. It was disempowering and we all just kinda chugged along after the first failure.

I can think of two things that I would do now that I've got a lot more experience with all this. First off, this was a failure long before we got our appeal to power shut down. We should have had better relations with Maggy right from the start. When she came on, we should have had a meeting and presented to her who we were, our jobs and our needs, and been really clear and direct about that. That alone could have cleared up any nasty surprises. Looking back, I can't believe we didn't do that. You have to communicate about things long before conflict arises. When your first contact is negative and then your second contact is negative, do you expect to be able to get anywhere?

The second thing I would do differently is to really engage with the youth in terms of creating solutions. We just let things fizzle and burn out; essentially, we excluded the youth from the process. Even if it led to them doing something crazy that would get us kicked out, it at least would have been under their power instead of using a strategy in which we stopped bringing them to negotiations. Now that I'm the Adult Coordinator of YIA, I see that this was an opportunity to actually have built an ally in the space (Maggy). It didn't have to get to that point. Yet once it did, we could have escalated our strategy instead of just burning out. To do something that rallied the larger supportive community around us would have been more confrontational to Draconi, but it would have proved our power and even built our own counter power to the building administrators.

I think this points out a larger contradiction in SJYD youth work. We can build groups that are very aware of power dynamics, but when we confront injustice in our communities, the consequences for oppressed youth of color can be very real. Organizing against the housing project in which these young people and their families live can have consequences. In this way, it was so important for us to have built alliances with Maggy, residents, families, and others to support us in our overall goals.

Unpacking the dilemma

Before analyzing the dilemma, it must first be acknowledged that this dilemma became so intense because YIA is situated within a SJYD framework. This is not to say that there are not tensions between youth and adults in traditional youth development programs. However, SJYD youth workers' dilemma cycles are unique in large part because they are generally working to challenge inequitable power relations.

Youth workers operating from a SJYD perspective consistently consider larger societal inequities and power relationships in their dilemma resolution process. This expanded understanding of what constitutes a "dilemma" transforms youth worker praxis by combining a focus upon the immediate needs and supportive development of youth with a focus on positively developing the place of young people in society as a whole. In many ways, a consideration of the macro dimensions of dilemmas may seem overwhelming. Layers of complex systemic and community issues certainly come into play for even the smallest dilemma. How can one youth worker afford to add more variables and worries to the mix, never mind tackling broad social change?

SJYD workers strive to analyze and take action on the levels that make practical sense in terms of the dilemma at hand, their own abilities, the directives of youth, and the degrees of youth participation and empowerment. They also have to make realistic decisions on what will impact both youth and community development positively. Rather than setting a bar so high that all dilemmas are a failure in regard to broad community social change, the inclusion of a broad ecological analysis provides workers with new spaces for intervention and action in youth work that value and balance community and personal development. We now apply the EDR model to Colin's dilemma.

Knowledge

Colin comes into this dilemma with rich personal knowledge from his experience creating a youth organization as a teenager. As a young person, when his community did not support him and his peer group, he worked to create the space they needed for their own self-determination. In college, this personal knowledge was validated through formal learning. He learns that his experience was not just an idiosyncratic one but, rather, represented an example of a grassroots effort forging democratic spaces of resistance against oppressive systems and structures.

Dilemma Resolution Cycle

Problem identification

At one level, the problem appears to be that Draconi management does not allow minors to be unsupervised in the Teen Zone. The problem could easily be resolved by Colin or Kim being present when the youth staff are working. Yet, YIA is founded on the principle of equitable youth-adult relationships. The youth staff have a job to do and they do it. Colin feels that they do not need him, Colin, who is only a few years older than the youth, to oversee their activities. So, rather than youth supervision being the problem, the group comes to the understanding that YIA's core mission is being threatened. The young people's efforts are being thwarted. This is not only undermining their productivity, but also their emerging activist identities.

Plan formulation

Colin is part of a decision to utilize their Batzaar structure to process and resolve these dilemmas. Through Batzaar, they decide to use a strategy that has worked in the past. They put together a professional presentation to explain YIA's mission and processes with hopes that this will help Maggy understand why young people often work beyond normal business hours.

Plan implementation

Colin and the young people are able to arrange for the presentation with Maggy; however, it does not yield the desired results. The group collectively decides on a strategy that refutes youth stereotypes, appeals to the Draconi sensibilities surrounding control and power, and maintains youth autonomy. However, unlike the experience with Lahn, this time the plan fails to impress Maggy and other managers. YIA appeals up the chain of command and eventually decides that youth being at the table may be hurting their efforts. As time goes on, adult staff meet with Draconi management, inadvertently disempowering the youth. The demoralization felt by both repeated defeat and decreasing youth participation impacts YIA's ability to innovate new strategies, leaving the group frustrated and angry but not effective.

Evaluation/reflection

A few years distance from the dilemma has given Colin time to reflect on where they went wrong with Maggy and the Draconi management. YIA's youth empowerment philosophy clashed with the views held by Draconi. Colin realizes that they grew frustrated, offended, angry, and disheartened. They only had one strategy, and when that failed, they simply refined the strategy by excluding youth and compromising their mission. Through reflection, Colin comes to realize—or to remember—that in order to effectively build power for youth activism, SJYD groups must also build communities that support and participate in this organizing as well.

REFLECTING ON PRACTICE:

What does Colin do well in this story? What strengths does he bring to youth work?

Where does Colin get stuck in this story? What keeps him from moving through the Dilemma Resolution Cycle?

What is happening in this case? What are the key factors Colin has to balance and weigh in order to achieve a positive outcome for the program and the youth?

In what ways can you relate to Colin's experience? Have you ever had your anger about injustices facing youth thwart your ability to work effectively with youth or on behalf of youth? What helped you push through?

How can youth workers help youth navigate rigid structures and conformities in life, such as workplace conventions, without taking away their decision-making and critical consciousness?

Summary

Did YIA not try hard enough? Did they not exert all their options and power? And if they didn't, how far should SJYD groups and organizations take their agendas for community change? The failure of both the collective organizing processes and the carefully constructed empowerment structures of YIA revealed disturbing limitations of real youth community engagement. Youth empowerment can be developed but faces long odds in communities in which the dominant framework is one of racist, classist, and ageist stereotypes. This clash over philosophies of power sent YIA, a fully functioning group, off the rails in both ideals and capacity. The reality is that as SJYD youth workers operate further away from the youth–centered microsystem, the legitimacy of youth power and agency rapidly diminishes (Roach et al., 2013).

This dilemma reveals how the SJYD framework and mindset is not in line with most of how society, especially adult society, thinks and acts. Plain and simple, young people cannot be trusted or held responsible. And while the YIA youth furiously attempted to change this notion, in the end they were forced to resort to adult exertion of power and subtle acts of resistance in order to get what they needed to continue their work. This example shows not only a pattern of SJYD principles slowly deteriorating in the face of a tough community dilemma, but also the value youth place on their own ability to navigate ecological systems. Colin's reflection indicates that effective SJYD youth worker praxis must move beyond establishing microsystem empowerment with youth by intentionally building community support for youth organizing before problems arise.

Digging deeper: applying the dilemma to your work

Activity 1: community mapping/power mapping

Social justice youth workers often find themselves focused heavily upon power dynamics in order to create spaces for youth to learn organizing skills and understand the role of identity and power in shaping community issues. However, this work may be limited if it does not proactively and intentionally build supportive community networks for youth organizing. This exercise focuses on a few skills youth workers can hone to develop supportive communities. Often this tool is used in community organizing at the start of a campaign. However, it is recommended here as a tool to map networks of people with whom you and your youth group want to build relationships, trust, and collaborative projects. Using Table 10.1 list relevant people and organizations in your community.

TABLE 10.1 Power mapping

Active allies (people who agree with you and are actively supportive)	Passive allies (people who agree but do not take action)	Neutral (people who don't know or care either way)	Passive opposition (people who disagree but aren't trying to stop you)	Active opposition (people who disagree and actively try to stop you)

This table is called your "Spectrum of Allies" and was developed by Daniel Hunter for the group Training for Change (Moore and Russell, 2011). The goal is not to move your active opposition to the active ally column, but to focus on moving passive opposition, neutral parties, and passive allies closer to being active allies. It is easy to mobilize and work with your active allies, but to work toward educating neutral groups, shifting the position of passive allies, or disrupting the status quo of active opposition takes much more.

- What active and passive allies do you already know?
- How often do you meet? How often do you collaborate or support one another's work?
- What neutral people or groups do you already know? Have you met with them?
- How can you make sure that your work is understood by neutral groups?
- Is there a way to communicate with passive opponents so as to shift them towards being a neutral party?

Make sure to do real solidarity work with your active and passive allies; supporting one another's projects goes a long way towards building a stronger community base. Make sure to meet with allies and neutral individuals to do one-to-one relational meetings with them.

Activity 2: one-to-ones (part two)

One-to-ones (or relational meetings) are one way to help build a more supportive community network for youth activism. In Chapter 3, we discuss the importance of youth workers using one-to-ones to build relationships with youth. Here, we recommend using them as an organizing tool for youth to build relationships with potential community partners and allies. These one-to-ones involve meeting with one other person to learn and share about each other's motivations to take action and be involved in the community. Meeting with people and listening to them talk about their primary focus within their community can help you and the youth in your group to understand the person, the many faces of the community you are in, and how to support one another in the work. One-to-ones help to build community networks that can grow movements, to bring to light new youth resources, and to proactively moderate conflict that may arise with time.

- Make a list of some of the people you want to build stronger relationships with in the community.
- Call them to set up brief meetings of 30 to 45 minutes and explain the purpose of a one-to-one.
- During these meetings, briefly introduce your work and have them explain their projects and work to you.
- Mostly spend this time listening to them and engaging them to understand their focus—what motivates them to do the work they do.

- Ask questions and go deeper into their answers, but don't pry or lead the conversation toward places they do not want to go.
- Share your motivations and commitments, and the reasons why you believe youth organizing is important to building strong communities.
- Keep it short and remember to thank them for their time!

Building these networks is necessary for understanding one another before conflict arises within the community. By establishing relationships between youth organizations and community institutions, we can change the climate in which youth organize as well as allow better navigation of obstacles within the community.

Activity 3: channeling anger into action

One of the biggest issues in this dilemma was the fact that the group lacked an overall strategy. Rather, they continued to use the same tactic of meeting with management over and over.

For this activity, sit down with your youth group and present a mock dilemma (or use the one from this chapter). First, establish with them what the end solution of the dilemma would be. Make sure that it is realistic for the context. Next, establish with the youth a strategy they may use to get there. What are the midpoint goals? What are the tactics? Discuss the difference between tactics and strategy. Do your tactics lead to smaller goals that will allow the group to obtain their bigger goals? What if one tactic does not work? What is the plan B? Plan C? By planning an overarching strategy ahead of time, YIA may have been able to change course instead of floundering. Plan with your group how they would create a larger strategy before obstacles arise.

References

Ginwright, S. and Cammarota, J. (2002). New terrain in youth development: The promise of a social justice approach. *Social Justice, 29*(4), 82–94.

Moore, H. and Russell, J. (2011). *Organizing cools the planet: Tools and reflections to navigate the climate crisis*. Oakland, CA: PM Press.

Roach, J., Wureta, E., and Ross, L. (2013). Dilemmas of practice in the ecology of emancipatory youth-adult partnerships. *International Journal of Child, Youth and Family Studies, 4*(3.1), 475–88.

11

CROSSCUTTING THEMES AND IMPLICATIONS FOR YOUTH WORKER PROFESSIONAL DEVELOPMENT

> Practical reasoning is deliberative, it takes into account local circumstances, it weighs tradeoffs, it is riddled with uncertainties, it depends on judgment, profits from wisdom, addresses particulars, it deals with contingencies, is iterative and shifts aims in process when necessary. Practical reasoning is the stuff of practical life. It is not the stuff of theoretical science. It is not enduring and it is not foundational. Its aim is to arrive at good but imperfect decisions with respect to particular circumstances.
>
> (Eisner, 2002: 375)

The dilemmas presented in this book are indeed both everyday and extraordinary. Youth workers recognize these as dilemmas they regularly face in their daily work with young people. They deal with navigating their role and forging relationships with youth, setting high expectations for youth while acknowledging the realities of their lives, handling risky incidents of violence and drug use, and keeping youth needs and well-being at the center of their practice. These dilemmas exemplify the ubiquitous tensions of relationships, values, and culture.

These tensions, while recurrent, are astonishingly challenging to navigate. As the Eisner quotation above suggests, they require wisdom about how to respond in particular situations that can never be equated with or reduced to general truths. In this chapter, we look across the dilemma stories and the knowledge and processes that the featured youth workers drew upon to address them. We organize this discussion around three crosscutting themes: roles and relationships, values and ethics, and culture and systems. We revisit the Ecological Dilemma Resolution (EDR) model as a tool to enhance novice and expert youth workers' ecological intelligence, and discuss ways that this model can be integrated into youth worker professional education.

Crosscutting themes

Roles and relationships

This book opens with the claim that the fundamental aim of youth work is to build trusting and mutually respectful relationships with young people. Scholars have suggested that "relationships are the backbone of effective youth work practice" (Young, 1999: 5). Likewise, most youth workers themselves would say that their work is all about relationships. But relationships are complex and can be challenging to negotiate. It is, therefore, no surprise that some of the stickiest dilemmas presented in this book involve navigating relationships. The different types of roles and relationships that youth workers establish serve distinct functions, from offering guidance and emotional support to providing authority and expertise (Walker, 2011). Across the dilemma scenarios presented in Chapters 3–10, the youth workers positioned themselves in different roles to respond to the needs of a given youth in a particular instance.

One set of dilemmas involves tension between relating to youth in a personal versus a professional way (Walker and Larson, 2006). On the one hand, youth workers are effective in their jobs when they can relate to youth in more informal, personal, and peer-like ways. A deeply relational approach can be helpful in building rapport, gaining trust, and motivating young people. In Chapter 3, Alexandra describes the turning point in her dilemma when she took a risk and shared her personal story with the youth. In Chapter 7, Katie outlines her efforts to establish a strong, caring relationship with a camper with special needs and how that bond was undermined by her organization's strict adherence to confidentiality procedures. In Chapter 9, Ricardo's established relationship with Anthony helped him read the dynamics underlying what could have been a particularly dangerous situation. As these instances illustrate, a personal relationship can help the youth worker understand the young person's perspective, motivations, and challenges.

On the other hand, youth workers also find themselves relating to youth from a professional stance. They may need to maintain youth's personal safety, ensure program activities are implemented, or represent the interests of the organization. In Chapter 6, Rebecca describes using her organization's Community Meeting process to address youth's violation of the program's code of conduct. Colin's dilemma, presented in Chapter 10, exemplifies the challenge of establishing youth-adult partnerships and working toward equitable or even emancipatory relationships when having to negotiate with a partner organization that did not share a Social Justice Youth Development mindset. Instances like these may require enforcing rules, considering accountability, and keeping an eye on issues and concerns that youth may not be thinking about.

Values and ethics

Ethical dilemmas can be among the hardest challenges faced by practitioners. They require a youth worker to decide what is right to do or how to be good in a given situation. "An ethical dilemma occurs when a person is confronted with a choice between two (or several) alternative courses of action, all of which may entail breaching some ethical principle or causing some potential harm" (Banks, 2010: 12). These important and anguishing situations require expeditious decision-making about value stances and issues of right and wrong.

Chapter 4 presents both Melinda's and Loren's struggles to determine whether to cut the very youth they are trying to reach; whether to consistently apply rules across all youth or to be more flexible and responsive to individual youth needs. In Chapter 5, Olivia describes a tension around reconciling family expectations and norms that are incongruent with her own hopes for the youth. In Chapter 7, Katie questions her organization's approach that privileged protecting client's confidentiality over informing and supporting staff. Her dilemma raises issues of rights, safety, trust, and privacy. Chapter 8 raises the question of whether a youth worker can or should counter the survival skills taught at home. Jessica asks, "how do you tell a youth that what their family is encouraging them to do is wrong, particularly when you as the youth worker can understand the logic underlying their actions because you were told the same thing?" Bronfenbrenner (1979) theorized that conditions for development are optimal when there is "value consensus" and communication between the different contexts in a young person's life. These scenarios illustrate the dilemmas that emerge when values consensus and communication across contexts are absent.

Culture and systems

Bronfrenbrenner's ecological model of human development outlines the interactions between youth and their environments. Young people do not exist in isolation; they are part of families and communities. Youth workers can better understand and support young people when they understand the relationships, contexts, influences, and experiences that affect their lives. In addition to the immediate settings, people, and events that impact a person, there are also systems that can exert power over them. Further, there are broad patterns of culture and society—economic and political structures—that influence a person's development, experiences, and choices.

A host of dilemmas involve tensions with worlds external to the program, including youth's outside lives, families, and cultures. The youth workers featured draw upon what Walker and Larson (2012) refer to as "ecological intelligence," or a deep, contextualized knowledge of youth culture and the systems that influence where young people live, learn, and play. For example, Chapters 8 and 9 present situations where the youth workers relied on their personal knowledge of gun and gang-related violence. Both youth workers' dilemmas in Chapter 4 illustrate how external factors affect young people's ability to fully participate in the youth programs. In Chapter 5, Olivia wrestles with multiple systems as she navigates how to support a young man coming out as gay to his parents. William, in Chapter 6, describes a dangerous situation where a program participant is involved in a fight outside of the program. He wrestles with whether and how to engage community partners like the police, the school, and community-based mediators. Across these cases, it is apparent that culture and context are important considerations.

Types of knowledge used to address dilemmas

How do youth workers figure out what to do in the face of such complex situations involving competing priorities and concerns? Chapter 2 outlines three types of knowledge that help practitioners navigate dilemmas of practice: propositional knowledge, practice knowledge, and personal knowledge. Next we examine how the youth workers featured in this book learned and applied these types of knowledge to their dilemma situations.

Propositional knowledge

Propositional knowledge—knowledge about youth development theory, research, and approaches to youth work—is the predominant learning outcome of most higher education and other nonprofit organizations' youth worker professional education in the United States. Youth workers with propositional knowledge about stages of child and adolescent development, theories of positive youth development, group dynamics, and program management are absolutely critical. Yet the ways youth workers in this book resolved their dilemmas suggest that propositional knowledge alone inadequately accounts for how they know what to do in the face of very challenging situations.

Do youth workers benefit from formal education, from grounding in youth development theory and principles of best practice? Does this make the work more "legitimate"? The youth workers featured in Chapters 3 and 10 draw upon their formal training in Social Justice Youth Development. For example, in college Alexandra majored in Sociology with a concentration on Youth Studies; this propositional knowledge influenced her social justice orientation. Yet for the most part, propositional knowledge is rarely mentioned in the cases; and if it is, it usually complicates rather than facilitates dilemma resolution. Formal education appears to be highly decontextualized from these youth worker's daily practice.

Practice knowledge

Practice knowledge or professional craft knowledge is gained from experience on the job. Practice knowledge is accumulated by doing the work over time and having opportunities to reflect-on-practice (Emslie, 2009; Hildreth and VeLure Roholt, 2013; Schön, 1990; Titchen and Ersser, 2001).

How do the youth workers featured in this volume benefit from on-the-job learning? Some of our cases illustrate how youth workers have drawn upon mentors. In Chapter 3, we see how after a particularly chaotic program session, Alexandra sought support from her mentor, Marc, who suggested she facilitate a listening activity with the group. In Chapter 5, when Olivia felt "in a little over my head," she sought support from her supervisor and youth worker colleagues in her network. Several of the youth workers featured also draw on on-the-job experience. Katie, in Chapter 7, developed a great deal of practice knowledge over the summer, which prepared her for her intensive, two-week session with Amy, a camper with special needs. Jessica, in Chapter 8, drew on networks she developed as a peer leader and staff, as well as knowledge she cultivated by putting herself "around people who I think I can learn something from."

Personal knowledge

The youth workers draw from their personal knowledge, knowledge that is the product of their own life and family experiences and events. Ross (2013) argues that youth worker expertise is based in part on personal knowledge derived from childhood neighborhood-based peer groups and participation in youth programs. Yet personal knowledge is not simply a matter of having had a collection of life experiences that may be similar to the youth's but, rather, a youth worker having made meaning of her own life story (Ross, 2013).

In some of the cases presented, the youth workers' personal knowledge was particularly relevant to how they responded to these complex dilemmas. The narratives in this book provide in-depth examples about how youth workers draw on personal knowledge. Jessica, Jacob, and Ricardo, the youth workers featured in Chapters 8 and 9, grew up in the same neighborhoods and attended similar youth programs as the youth they now serve. These experiences provided them with the knowledge to navigate dangerous neighborhoods, to "code switch" when in different groups and settings, and to negotiate complex family and peer relationships that both encourage and discourage getting ahead and moving away, as well as an expanded repertoire for thinking and acting from non-family mentors at youth programs. This knowledge helped them to balance the needs of the young people involved in violent activities with the safety and well-being of other youth and staff in the programs.

Practitioner expertise

All these types of knowledge collectively contribute to practitioner expertise. Practitioner expertise involves not just knowing *about* but knowing *how*: it involves knowledge and skills for both understanding and action. Further, it involves practical *know-how* or making sound, ethical choices in particular situations. Practitioner expertise is the ability to integrate and apply knowledge, skills, and judgment in practice. It is more than the demonstration of competencies; it is the ability to orchestrate multiple competencies into a full range of behaviors necessary for effective practice.

Implications for youth worker professional development

How do youth workers develop these types of knowledge that are used to address dilemmas of practice? Practitioner expertise is earned through prolonged practice

(Baizerman, 2009). It is acquired through experience and developed through habit. Yet veteran practitioners can go stale on a job from doing it in rote ways year after year. In fact, years of experience is a poor predictor of performance (Marsh, 2007). The research on expertise across a variety of fields suggests that beyond sheer years of experience or even natural ability, it is ongoing "deliberate practice" with feedback that matters in developing and maintaining expertise (Ericsson *et al.*, 2006). Deliberate practice is defined as appropriately challenging tasks that are chosen with the goal of improving a particular skill. We learn when we have ongoing opportunities to engage with the full range of challenges associated with our practice and receive authentic feedback. In other words, it's not about going through the motions, but having ongoing opportunities to work at addressing some of the most difficult problems in one's field with coaching, questioning, and critical reflection (Walker and Walker, 2011).

Having a skilled youth worker workforce is critical. Studies consistently suggest that the expertise of front-line staff is the most central factor in program impact (Hirsch *et al.*, 2011; McLaughlin *et al.*, 1994; Vandell *et al.*, 2015). Yet a concern in the field of youth development is that many front-line staff begin with little training and develop their professional skills in isolation. They have limited opportunity to reflect, read research, or learn from peers or expert practitioners (Walker and Walker, 2011). In this section, we discuss the role of documenting and sharing both dilemmas and strategies for effectively responding to them. Further, we discuss how the EDR model can be utilized to foster deliberate practice in youth worker professional education.

Documenting dilemmas

Dilemmas are inherent and inevitable; uncertainty, doubt, and not-knowing are normal features of youth work (Anderson-Nathe, 2010). The work of running a program and facilitating youth development is more complex and multidimensional than is generally appreciated (Larson *et al.*, forthcoming). Therefore, it is important to share our dilemma stories, to recognize that others have similar struggles, and to feel affirmed rather than alienated. The writing and use of case examples, as done in the previous chapters, is particularly useful for understanding the range of dilemmas front-line staff face in their work (Banks and Nohr, 2003; Larson *et al.*, forthcoming). Dilemma-based cases can be used in professional development in a variety of ways. Participants can analyze the scenarios, individually or as a group, to identify considerations at play as well as to generate possible responses.

Another strength and contribution of the previous chapters is that they provide practitioner perspectives, voices that are too often lacking in scholarly literature. Their dilemma cases illustrate how youth workers are continually experimenting, learning from, reflecting on, and improving what they do. A problem in the youth development field is that much of this hard-earned knowledge about daily practice is not documented, systemized, and made available in centralized sources (Larson *et al.*, forthcoming).

Documenting strategies

Beyond documenting the array of dilemmas encountered in practice, it is essential that we better understand the variety of strategies that effective practitioners employ to address these challenges (Larson *et al.*, forthcoming). Strategies include principles and guidelines they use, considerations they weigh, resources they draw upon, and skills they employ to address dilemmas. These might be proactive strategies to avoid a dilemma as well as reactive strategies to navigate dilemmas that occur. We outline four strategies that the youth workers featured in Chapters 3–10 employed.

Craft youth-centered responses

One crosscutting feature of the strategies employed by expert youth workers is that they craft youth-centered responses. Larson and Walker (2010) identify four dimensions of youth-centered responses: 1) engaging directly with youth, 2) turning the dilemma into an opportunity for youth's development, 3) incorporating youth into the solution or response to the situation, and 4) advocating on behalf of youth as well as teaching youth to advocate for themselves. They found that experts reported significantly more youth-centered responses than novices, and that experts more often described responses that converted the dilemmas into opportunities for youth development (Walker and Larson, 2012).

In Chapter 5, Olivia is very intentional about keeping youth and their needs at the center, as her mirror metaphor implies. She sees her role as supporting youth, and she also recognizes the importance of her own self-care in this process. In Chapter 4, Loren puts the youth struggles at the center of her decision to restructure the program to better meet their needs. In Chapter 10, Colin reflects on his program's social justice principles and the importance of a youth-centered response by recognizing the need to create teachable moments and engage the young people in responding to the dilemma at hand. Being youth-centered is related to propositional knowledge about the foundational principles of positive youth development. Knowing how to keep youth at the center requires deliberative practice.

Seek support from mentors and supervisors

Youth workers need to feel supported by people they respect and who have actual work experience in the field. It is particularly helpful to draw upon the knowledge and experiences of mentors and supervisors who have been doing youth work in the trenches (Wood *et al.*, 2015). In Chapter 3, Alexandra acknowledges that one of her major turning points came when she took the advice of her mentor, Marc, to facilitate a listening activity with the group. In Chapter 9, Jacob draws on what he learned from his mentor, Bobby, about diffusing a potentially dangerous situation: "the real guy you've got to watch is the guy who moves in silence." In Chapter 10, Colin's first year at YIA resembles an apprenticeship in which he learns to be a social justice youth worker by watching and supporting Kim, a more experienced coworker. These cases show how consulting with a mentor is one way to develop practice knowledge.

Think on your feet

Youth workers must make decisions about courses of action in dynamic, ambiguous, and multidimensional situations (Fook *et al.*, 2000). As Kahneman and Klein describe for other professional fields, "experts are expected to successfully attain vaguely defined goals in the face of uncertainty, time pressures, high stakes, team and organizational constraints, [and] shifting conditions" (2009: 516). The youth workers featured in Chapters 6, 8, and 9 demonstrate how their personal and practice knowledge allows them to think on their feet and read and respond to very complex, high-stress, and nuanced situations. In crafting their response, their personal knowledge allows them to "code switch" and take into account considerations from the culture of the street and the perspectives of community members as well as from the culture and perspectives of the youth organizations involved. Alternately, in Chapter 3, we see how novice youth workers routinely struggle with the ability to think on their feet. Thinking on one's feet is a blend of personal and practice knowledge; it is informed by experience and honed with practice.

Consider organizational perspectives

Youth programs are situated within organizations, and organizational priorities and policies can both help and hinder what front-line youth workers consider to be in the best interest of the young people. In Chapter 8, Jessica deliberates with her coworkers and supervisors about their organization's reputation and partners' perceptions as well as how disciplinary and safety protocols should guide their work. Loren and Melinda in Chapter 4 illustrate that there are times when enforcing rules is most important, as well as times when making accommodations is most appropriate. Upon reflection, Melinda comes to see how enforcing program rules consistently holds youth to high standards whereas Loren adapts the program rather than strictly adhering to rules. In Chapter 6, William laments not having known or relied on his organization's protocols to support himself in handling a dangerous situation. In Katie's case, presented in Chapter 7, she felt the organization's priority on privacy—while well intentioned—impeded her efforts to support the youth. In Chapter 5, Olivia rejects her organization's directive to refer a youth to another agency. Being aware of organizational rules and procedures is propositional knowledge, but knowing how and when to apply and flex those policies requires activating practice and personal knowledge.

Developing knowledge

Dilemma-based case examples can be used to help novice youth workers identify value choices, consider multiple perspectives, and generate creative responses to nuanced and dynamic situations. Practitioners feel most challenged, stretched, and engaged when dealing with real-world situations like those presented in this book (Endsley, 2006). Next we outline several approaches to using dilemma-based cases for professional development of youth worker expertise.

Create networks of support with colleagues and mentors

It is essential that youth workers have the opportunity to discuss dilemmas in a climate of safety and support (Anderson-Nathe, 2010). We need more places where youth workers can come together to discuss their work and learn from one another. It is particularly useful for practitioners to explore these cases with their peers so they can engage in dialogue and reflection that stimulates new ways to approach their work. Youth workers highly value a cohort of peers with whom they can share and learn, develop professionally, and be encouraged to think in new ways. They appreciate a reciprocal learning environment where they are learning from one another.

Build opportunities for reflection and dialogue that cultivate ecological intelligence

These narratives demonstrate that there is considerable benefit in analysis of dilemma scenarios to become more aware of issues and more intentional about responses. Personal introspection with a dilemma-focused learning journal is one way to encourage reflection. It forces oneself to stop and think and can help one make sense of feelings and patterns. Banks and Nohr (2003) illustrate how Socratic dialogue—a method for questioning and investigating our thinking and feeling and assumptions—can help transform practitioners' ways of thinking about themselves and their work. Practitioners learn from participating in reflective spaces in which they are invited to articulate, discuss, and examine the experiences and thinking they do every day—a process that helps them become more explicit about the underlying assumptions and theories of practice that guide their actions (Spillane et al., 2002). Through activities like collective deliberation of case studies, Socratic dialogue, and mind-mapping of dilemmas, youth workers can enhance their skills in attending to the complexity of real-world practice and develop the capacity to address diverse considerations while keeping youth needs at the center. The "Unpacking the dilemma" and "Digging deeper: applying the dilemma to your work" sections in Chapters 3–10 provide specific tools for reflection, dialogue, and action.

Apply the Ecological Dilemma Resolution model

Chapter 2 presents the EDR model, a four-stage Dilemma Resolution Cycle that guides youth workers to utilize reflective practices to deliberatively activate their personal, practice, and propositional knowledge for the purpose of cultivating ecological intelligence. More than *learning about* effective practice, the EDR advances a "dilemma-based pedagogy" that helps *improve* youth work practice. Guided, systematic analysis of dilemma cases assists youth workers to develop patterns of thought needed to conduct comprehensive yet rapid analysis of dilemma situations when they are on the job.

What are the implications of this model for training? How can this model help people figure out what to do when facing a dilemma? What questions might one ask oneself at each stage? Consider some of the questions we pose in the "Reflecting on practice" boxes, as well as those from Banks and Nohr (2003); for example:

- To appraise the situation, you might consider: What considerations (concerns, priorities) did you have in this situation? What were the different things at stake? Whose interests were at stake? What did you weigh or think about when deciding what to do? Also, what were the facts?
- To formulate a plan, you might consider: How will your response address the considerations? Which considerations "trump" other things or drive your response? Are there underlying values or goals that influenced your decision? What prior experiences influence how you handled this decision? What resources are available to you?
- To implement a plan, you might consider: How will you carry out your decision? Who do you need to involve?
- To reflect and take stock on how you carried out your plan, you might consider: How successful do you think your response was? With the benefit of hindsight, was there anything you might have done differently?

Working through a staged process like the EDR model can help one break down and frame a dilemma situation, sometimes opening up new possibilities. It can help orient us to and take into account different dimensions of the dilemma. While it does not automatically provide the "correct" solution, it pushes one to systematically analyze the situation from different angles and to address the situation more deliberately. It can help strip the situation of emotionally charged tensions and help one avoid impulsive responses.

Concluding thoughts

Everyday youth work is rife with extraordinarily complex dilemmas. Creating and sustaining conditions for young people to develop is not straightforward, and the expertise required goes far beyond common sense or what can be found in a textbook. To fully understand, recognize, and elevate the significance of youth work, we need more practice-based research that documents and builds theory about its complexity from the practitioners' point of view. Further, we need professional development that accounts for and fosters reflection on the complex reality of everyday youth work practice.

References

Anderson-Nathe, B. (2010). *Youth workers, stuckness, and the myth of supercompetence.* New York: Routledge.

Baizerman, M. (2009). Deepening understanding of managing evaluation. In D. W. Compton and M. Baizerman (Eds.), *Managing program evaluation: Towards explicating a professional practice. New directions for evaluation, No. 121.* San Francisco, CA: Jossey-Bass (pp. 87–98).

Banks, S. (2010). Ethics and the youth worker. In S. Banks (Ed.), *Ethical issues in youth work.* 2nd edition. New York: Routledge (pp. 3–23).

Banks, S. and Nohr, K. (2003). *Teaching practical ethics for the social professions.* Copenhagen, Denmark: FESET.

Bronfenbrenner, U. (1979). *The ecology of human development: Experiments by nature and design.* Cambridge, MA: Harvard University Press.

Eisner, E. W. (2002). From episteme to phronesis to artistry in the study and improvement of teaching. *Teaching and Teacher Education, 18*(4), 375–85.

Emslie, M. (2009). Researching reflective practice: A case study of youth work education. *Reflective Practice, 10*(4), 417–27.

Endsley, M. (2006). Expertise and situation awareness. In K. A. Ericsson, N. Charness, P. J. Feltovich, and R. R. Hoffman (Eds.), *Cambridge handbook of expertise and expert performance: Its development, organization and content.* Cambridge, UK: Cambridge University Press (pp. 633–52).

Ericsson, K. A., Charness, N., Feltovich, P. J., and Hoffman, R. R. (Eds.). (2006). *Cambridge handbook of expertise and expert performance: Its development, organization and content.* Cambridge, UK: Cambridge University Press.

Fook, J., Ryan, M., and Hawkins, L. (2000). *Professional expertise: Practice, theory and education for working in uncertainty.* London, UK: Whiting and Birch.

Hildreth, R. and VeLure Roholt, R. (2013). Teaching and training civic youth workers: Creating spaces for reciprocal civic and youth development. In R. VeLure Roholt, M. Baizerman, and R. Hildreth (Eds.), *Civic youth work: Co-creating democratic youth spaces.* Chicago: Lyceum Books (pp. 151–9).

Hirsch, B. J., Deutsch, N. L., and DuBois, D. L. (2011). *After-school centers and youth development: Case studies in success and failure.* New York: Cambridge University Press.

Kahneman, D. and Klein, G. (2009). Conditions for intuitive expertise: A failure to disagree. *American Psychologist, 64*(6), 515–26.

Larson, R. and Walker, K. (2010). Dilemmas of practice: Challenges to program quality encountered by youth program leaders. *American Journal of Community Psychology, 45*(3–4), 338–49.

Larson, R., Walker, K., Rusk, N., and Diaz, L. B. (forthcoming). Understanding youth development from the practitioner's point of view: A call for research on effective practice. *Applied Developmental Science.*

McLaughlin, M., Irby, M., and Langman, J. (1994). *Urban sanctuaries: Neighborhood organizations in the lives and futures of inner-city youth.* San Francisco, CA: Jossey-Bass.

Marsh, H. W. (2007). Do university teachers become more effective with experience? A multilevel growth model of students' evaluations of teaching over 13 years. *Journal of Educational Psychology, 99*(4), 775–90.

Ross, L. (2013). Urban youth workers' use of "personal knowledge" in resolving complex dilemmas of practice. *Child & Youth Services, 34*(3), 267–89.

Schön, D. (1990). *Educating the reflective practitioner: Toward a new design for teaching and learning in the professions.* San Francisco: Jossey Bass.

Spillane, J. P., Reiser, B. J., and Reimer, T. (2002). Policy implementation and cognition: Reframing and refocusing implementation research. *Review of Educational Research, 72*(3), 387–431.

Titchen, A. and Ersser, S. (2001). Explicating, creating and validating professional craft knowledge. In J. Higgs and A. Titchen (Eds.), *Practice knowledge and expertise in the health professions*. Oxford: Butterworth-Heinemann (pp. 48–56).

Vandell, D. L., Larson, R. W., Mahoney, J. L., and Watts, T. W. (2015). Children's organized activities. In M. H. Bornstein, T. Leventhal, and R. Lerner (Eds.), *Handbook of child psychology and developmental science: Ecological settings and processes in developmental systems. Vol. 4.* 7th edition. New York: Wiley (pp. 305–44).

Walker, J. and Walker, K. (2011). Establishing expertise in an emerging field. In D. Fusco (Ed.), *Advancing youth work: Current trends, critical questions*. New York: Routledge (pp. 39–51).

Walker, K. (2011). The multiple roles that youth development program leaders adopt with youth. *Youth & Society, 43*(2), 635–55.

Walker, K. and Larson, R. (2006). The dilemmas of youth work: Balancing the personal and professional. *New Directions for Youth Development, 112,* 109–18.

Walker, K. and Larson, R. (2012). Youth worker reasoning about dilemmas encountered in practice: Expert-novice differences. *Journal of Youth Development, 7*(1), 5–23.

Wood, J., Westwood, S., and Thompson, G. (2015). *Youth work: Preparation for practice.* London: Routledge.

Young, K. (1999). *The art of youth work.* Lyme Regis: Russell House.

INDEX